D0220786

APPLIED PHONETICS WORKBOOK

A Systematic Approach to Phonetic Transcription

Third Edition

APPLIED PHONETICS WORKBOOK

A Systematic Approach to Phonetic Transcription

Third Edition

Harold T. Edwards, Ph.D.
Alvin L. Gregg, Ph.D.
Department of Communicative Disorders and Sciences
Wichita State University
Wichita, Kansas

THOMSON
DELMAR LEARNING™
Australia • Canada • Mexico • Singapore • Spain • United Kingdom • United States

THOMSON
DELMAR LEARNING

Applied Phonetics Workbook: A Systematic Approach to Phonetic Transcription, Third Edition
by Harold T. Edwards and Alvin L. Gregg

Executive Director:
William Brottmiller

Executive Editor:
Cathy L. Esperti

Developmental Editor:
Darcy M. Scelsi

Editorial Assistant:
Maria D'Angelico

Executive Marketing Manager:
Dawn F. Gerrain

Channel Manager:
Jennifer McAvey

Marketing Coordinator:
Kim Lourinia

Production Manager:
Barbara A. Bullock

Art and Design Coordinator:
Connie Lundberg-Watkins

Production Coordinator:
Jessica Peterson

Project Editor:
David Buddle

Printed in the United States of America
1 2 3 4 5 6 XXX 07 06 05 04 03 02

For more information, contact Delmar Learning, 5 Maxwell Drive, Clifton Park, NY 12065. Or find us on the World Wide Web at http://www.delmarlearning.com

Library of Congress Catalog Card Number
2002034829

ISBN 0-7693-0261-0

Contents

For the Student

As you will soon see, the regular spelling of English does not represent the sounds of English adequately. Therefore, a special phonetic alphabet is needed. Such an alphabet has been devised by the International Phonetic Association (IPA), and is known as the International Phonetic Alphabet (also IPA). By using this workbook, you will learn to use a form of it to transcribe English speech. Phonetic transcription is a permanent record of speech using symbols that represent the actual sounds as spoken. This workbook is designed to enable you to learn to transcribe through a series of logical and systematic steps.

Initially, the beginner might be overwhelmed by the number of new symbols to be learned. Yet many of the IPA symbols represent sounds commonly associated with their counterparts in the English alphabet. For a few of the IPA symbols corresponding to English letters, you will have to learn a new sound value. Obviously, the remaining symbols must be learned. In this workbook, a manageable number of symbols is introduced at one time for study and practice. In each group of symbols, there will be some to be learned or relearned and some that are familiar. The order in which the sounds are presented in this book reflects many years of helping students learn to transcribe speech. A mix of consonants and vowels is presented in each section to balance the task of learning to transcribe speech and make your effort more interesting. Frequently used symbols tend to be introduced before rarely used symbols. Symbols or sounds that conflict with other symbols or sounds are not introduced together in the same section.

You should keep in mind that your ultimate task is learning each symbol along with its corresponding sound. To accomplish this, you will need to use the flashcards provided with this workbook, as described in Section 1. If you have a knowledge of the sound-symbol correspondences introduced in each section, you will be able to make more efficient progress in attaining your goal. Your initial class transcriptions will probably come from exercises in this book and will be based on sounds that have previously been introduced. After you become proficient with phonetic transcription, your teacher will want you to transcribe words and phrases not found in this workbook.

Each section in the first part of this workbook begins with Learning Activities that will help you to understand the sounds and symbols you will learn. For these you will also need the accompanying text, *Applied Phonetics: The Sounds of American English*. The Learning Activities are followed by Transcription Exercises that develop your ability to transcribe. In subsequent sections, other sets of symbols are introduced with their Learning Activities and Transcription Exercises. In this way, you are given a chance to build your skills, a little at a time, with graded exercises that help you to avoid common transcription pitfalls.

The compact disks included with this workbook provide an additional source for learning and practice. Audio-transcription Activities have been provided so that you may develop your ear for hearing and transcribing speech sounds in various contexts.

An eventual source of confusion for anyone who transcribes speech phonetically is that authorities do not always agree about which symbols to use or their exact form. There are several different phonetic alphabets in use in the English-speaking world. Even when the same system is used, there is some disagreement among teachers and authors about special details of transcription. In this workbook there are notes about some of these variant forms and practices. In such cases, students should transcribe as their teachers instruct. For anyone who desires to read research in the area of phonetics, however, it is necessary to have some knowledge of the variations found among transcribers of speech.

This workbook provides tips on how to transcribe with a minimum of error. You will want to make a special point of reading and understanding both the descriptive material and the instructions before starting the activities and exercises in each section.

Exercises are also provided on the different dialects of American English. You should first learn to hear and transcribe the sounds of your own dialect. Then you will be able to hear and transcribe the sounds of other dialects more readily.

Finally, there is the question of how carefully transcribers should go into detail in making transcriptions. Should the tiniest sound difference be captured by a special symbol or *diacritic* (a marking that is used with a standard symbol to alter its corresponding sound)? Or will minor differences be lumped together so that only the most important linguistic features are reflected in the transcription? When we try to capture minute differences in pronunciation, we make a *narrow* transcription, but when our interest is to record major sound differences, a *broad* transcription will suffice. Some aspects of American English can only be treated by conventions that are considered "narrow" in scope, so the student cannot avoid learning special symbols and diacritical marks from the beginning. Therefore, the goal of most transcribers is to aim for some point between the tedious narrow transcription and the sometimes misleading broad transcription.

Phonetic transcription is not a way of respelling English words, but of training your ear for all kinds of decision making. As you develop as a transcriber, you will begin to hear variations in your own speech more accurately as well as subtle variations in the speech of others. For clinical phoneticians, a lasting benefit will be the ability to hear and understand deviations in speech, knowledge that will ultimately lead to appropriate clinical procedures.

This workbook is organized in two parts. Part I will acquaint you with the sounds of American English, their phonetic symbols, their major dialect variations, transcription principles, and use of the alphabet of the IPA as generally interpreted by American phoneticians to transcribe speech. Once again, to make complete and efficient use of the *Applied Phonetics Workbook: A Systematic Approach to Phonetic Transcription*, you will also need the accompanying text, *Applied Phonetics: The Sounds of American English*, which contains the information necessary to complete the Learning Activities in addition to specialized information on each of the sounds of American English.

Part II deals with advanced phonetic transcription, including the transcription of connected speech, dialect differences, non-native speech, and disordered speech. You will find that the exercises in Part II will add enjoyment to your work and will not only give you an opportunity to put into practice everything you learned in Part I, but extend your ability to a higher level.

The appendixes found at the end of this workbook are important. You will use them to complete some of the exercises and to check your answers to ensure that you are transcribing accurately.

Before long you will become skillful in transcribing speech phonetically and will develop a deeper appreciation of American English and its sounds. By consistent, systematic endeavor, you will find phonetic transcription interesting and useful. In short, you will have become a phonetician!

Acknowledgments

This text was written to assist students in becoming (a) knowledgeable about the sounds of American English and (b) accurate transcribers of speech. If we have succeeded, it has been due to the high level of positive criticism that students provided as these materials were tested in the classroom. Several hundred students have helped to shape the substance and the form of this book, and to each we owe a debt of gratitude.

In addition, colleagues have critically evaluated our ideas, helped in developing some of the exercises, reviewed the manuscript, and tested the materials in their classrooms. These include Martha Boose, Collette Coleman, Alice Dyson, Mary Gordon, Barbara Hodson, Julie Scherz, Carl Wohlgemuth, Abby Cameron, and Lori Hartnett.

Our hope is that we have understood and implemented correctly the valuable assistance offered by everyone who has given life to this workbook and its accompanying text.

PART I
MASTERING THE BASICS

SECTION 1

The Phonetic Alphabet: An Overview

The purpose of this introductory section is to acquaint you with the alphabet that will be used throughout this workbook. You will soon discover that in phonetic transcription, the difficult task initially is *not* learning the symbols but rather making the *sound-symbol* association—that is, training your "ear" to hear the form of speech rather than the content of speech. The first part of this process is to become aware of the magnitude of the task.

■ The Phonetic Alphabet

Fortunately, many of the symbols used in the alphabet of the International Phonetic Association (IPA) are already familiar to speakers of English. Because symbols like /p/, /b/, and /m/ represent the same sounds in both the English and IPA alphabets, new sound associations do not have to be learned for them. Nevertheless, the English alphabet is not adequate for the phonetic transcription. For example, the most frequent vowel sound in spoken English (called the *schwa* or reduced vowel, sometime written *uh*, and transcribed /ə/) has no letter to represent it in the alphabet. In fact, there are only five letters—a, e, i, o, and u—for almost all of our vowel sounds, and all five of them sometimes represent the schwa sound, as in *a*blaze, rem*e*dy, *i*nitial, the*o*retical, and radi*u*m. Anyone who has spent countless hours learning to spell knows that our current alphabet poses problems that are compounded when we want to transcribe actual speech.

From the 26 Letters, We Need More

Examine the letters of the English alphabet:

a b c d e f g h i j k l m n o p q r s t u v w x y z

We have already seen that English has a reduced vowel sound (schwa) with no letter to represent it. Moreover, in spelling, each of the letters for the vowel sounds—a, e, i, o, u—may represent different sounds. For example, the letter *o* is pronounced differently in *go*, *got*, *woman*, and *women*. Because there are at least 13 more vowel sounds in English than there are letters for vowels, we must give a specific sound to each of these five vowel symbols, and then assign new symbols to the remaining vowel sounds. With the five vowel letters removed for later consideration, our alphabet has shrunk to 21 letters:

b c d f g h j k l m n p q r s t v w x y z

But of these, the *c, q*, and *x* may be written with other letters as in "sir*k*us" (circus), "*k*wack" (quack), "bo*ks*" (box), and "*z*ylophone" (xylophone); in addition, the founders of the International Phonetic Association decided to use /j/ for the consonant sound represented in the alphabet by *y* in *you*. Therefore, by omitting the *c, q, x*, and *y*, we are left with:

b d f g h k l m n p r s t v w z and /j/

What this means is that you already know 16 or 17 of the symbols used for the consonants in the phonetic alphabet.

In *For the Student*, you learned the difference between a *broad* transcription—record of major sound differences—and a *narrow* transcription—a record of particular sound differences. Broad transcriptions are usually placed within virgules or slashes / /, whereas transcriptions done to show more phonetic detail are sometimes placed in brackets [ ]. We recommend that you *remember* these conventions. However, to keep your transcriptions easier to read, *do not use virgules or brackets* in this workbook unless your teacher specifies otherwise. Individual sounds, of course, should be written within slashes, for example, /p/, when it is necessary to differentiate them from alphabet letters.

Transcription Exercise 1.1

Provide the consonant symbol(s) that you already know for the missing sounds. The vowel is already transcribed. Use a sheet of paper to cover the answers, and then uncover the answers to check your work. Make sure that your answers resemble in every way the handwritten examples that are provided. Become familiar with Appendix A of this book so that you can check your written work. Remember to use only these symbols: b d f g h k l m n p r s t v w z and /j/. Also note that the phonetic symbol for *g* is /g/.

	Fill in the Blanks			Written Form
Example: a male child	b ɔɪ	boy	/bɔɪ/	bɔɪ
1. Chess is a ____	_ e _	game	/gem/	gem
2. An animal that barks	_ ɔ _	dog	/dɔg/	dɔg
3. A ____ of gum	_ _ ɪ _	stick	/stɪk/	stɪk
4. Used in baseball to hit	_ æ _	bat	/bæt/	bæt
5. In baseball, a home ____	_ ʌ _	run	/rʌn/	rʌn
6. Pronoun for the other speaker	_ u	you	/ju/	ju
7. Once around a track	_ æ _	lap	/læp/	læp
8. An adult male	_ æ _	man	/mæn/	mæn
9. A shopping ____	_ ɪ _ _	list	/lɪst/	lɪst
10. A device for regulating the flow through a pipe	_ æ _ _	valve	/vælv/	vælv
11. labor, toil	_ ɝ _	work	/wɝk/	wɝk
12. Between 3 and 5	_ ɔ _	four	/fɔr/	fɔr
13. Front of the head	_ e _	face	/fes/	fes
14. Postal ____ Code	_ ɪ _	zip	/zɪp/	zɪp
15. ____ and roll	_ ɑ _	rock	/rɑk/	rɑk
16. A sound made by a cat	_ _ u	mew	/mju/	mju

17. Plural of "key"	_ i _	keys	/kiz/	kiz
18. Plural of "goose"	_ i _	geese	/gis/	gis
19. It produces light	_ æ _ _	lamp	/læmp/	laemp
20. A squeaking sound	_ _ i _	creak	/krik/	krik

Using the Compact Disks That Accompany This Workbook

Students make faster progress in learning to transcribe speech phonetically if they can hear actual examples of the speech sounds—in isolation, words, and phrases—their variations in different phonetic environments (their interactions with other speech sounds), and how they change across dialects. To this end, three compact disks (CDs) have been prepared for use, along with the Learning Activities and Transcription Exercises in this workbook. Continued use of the CDs will make learning to transcribe speech more efficient and enjoyable.

Each CD is organized into tracks and each Audio-Activity occupies a separate track. By pausing or replaying the track, additional practice can be obtained. Instructions for each Audio-Activity are provided, along with space for completing each activity in this workbook. In addition, the answers for each activity are given, but should be covered during the presentation of the audio material. In this way, immediate feedback can be obtained on your progress in transcribing actual speech. We have tried to provide sufficient time on the activity track for you to transcribe each item before the next is presented. If you need additional time, however, use the pause button on your CD player.

The flash cards that accompany this workbook are needed for some Audio-Activities. The number on each card will assist in organizing them for use in these activities. You should proceed through the Learning Activities, Transcription Exercises, and Audio-Activities in the order presented to make your learning incremental and systematic.

There are four different speakers on the CDs (in alphabetical order): Drs. Harold Edwards, Alvin Gregg, Julie Scherz, and Kathy Strattman. Other samples were provided by non-native speakers of English and children with various phonological delays.

Audio-Activity 1.1. Making Sound-Symbol Associations from the English Alphabet: Consonants (CD 1, Track 1)

In this activity, the first for which you will use the CDs that accompany this workbook, you will match sounds and symbols using the letters of the alphabet—phonetic symbols that you already know. Write one symbol for each sound that you hear. For example, you will hear, "Transcribe /pɪ/ as in *pit.*" We will add the vowel /ɪ/ to the sound so that you can hear it better. The symbol that you write in the space provided will be the *first sound* in the key word that you hear. There are 22 items. For items 19 to 22, be sure to use the adapted symbols /g/ and /j/ as appropriate. Cover the answers, then check your work.

		Answers	
1. _______	2. _______	/p/	/d/
3. _______	4. _______	/m/	/s/
5. _______	6. _______	/f/	/w/
7. _______	8. _______	/l/	/f/
9. _______	10. _______	/b/	/k/
11. _______	12. _______	/h/	/v/
13. _______	14. _______	/r/	/b/
15. _______	16. _______	/n/	/z/
17. _______	18. _______	/t/	/p/
19. _______	20. _______	/g/	/j/
21. _______	22. _______	/g/	/j/

The Vowel Sounds

Let us return to the five vowel letters from the alphabet: a, e, i, o, u. As we have said previously, it is necessary to assign a consistent sound to each symbol. It is more difficult for the beginning transcriber to learn what sound is reassigned to these familiar letters than to learn a new symbol that is associated with a particular sound. Try to discover what sound is assigned to each of the five alphabet letters in the next exercise.

Transcription Exercise 1.2

Using only the five alphabet symbols for the vowel sounds—ɑ, e, i, o, and u (notice how the symbol for *a* is written, /ɑ/)—determine which is the most appropriate answer for the clue that is provided. Cover the answers and then check your guesses with the answers.

		Printed Answers	Written Answers
1. The doctor says, "Open wide and say ____."	______	/ɑ/	a
2. An exclamation of disbelief "____, really?"	______	/o/	o
3. An exclamation of enjoyment, often represented by "Ooooooo!"	______	/u/	u
4. A partial scream, as when a mouse is seen unexpectedly.	______	/i/	i
5. The usual pronunciation of the letter *a*.	______	/e/	e

Transcription Exercise 1.3

Now transcribe these simple words, paying attention to the vowel sound in each. Cover the answers before you begin. Then check your work.

		Answers
1. hot	______	/hɑt/
2. hate	______	/het/
3. hoot	______	/hut/
4. heat	______	/hit/
5. hoe	______	/ho/

Audio-Activity 1.2. Making Sound-Symbol Associations from the English Alphabet: Vowels (CD 1, Track 2)

Listen to these 10 words containing examples of the 5 vowel symbols from the alphabet and transcribe the appropriate symbol in the spaces provided. See Transcription Exercise 1.2 and study flashcard 38 for the way to write the *a* letter phonetically. Cover the answers before you begin.

		Answers	
1. ______	2. ______	/e/	/ɑ/
3. ______	4. ______	/i/	/o/
5. ______	6. ______	/u/	/o/
7. ______	8. ______	/u/	/ɑ/
9. ______	10. ______	/i/	/e/

The "New" Symbols

Now that you know how to make sound-symbol associations, we will introduce all the other basic symbols for the vowel and consonant sounds that you will need in transcribing English speech. However, we will wait until later in this text to drill them in detail. At this point, try to become familiar with each one. A space is provided for you to transcribe each key word. Following that is another word for you to transcribe, which is almost like the key word. Once again, you can check your transcription with the answer. At this time, do not be concerned with dialect differences. Your instructor will help you to hear any differences between your own dialect and the one used for some of these words. It is important that your symbols look *exactly* like the written form; this is especially true for the last four vowel symbols that require the addition of a slur /‿/.

The Vowel Symbols

Symbol Printed Form	Symbol Written Form						
/ɪ/	/ɪ/	as in hit	/hɪt/	_______	bit	_______	/bɪt/
/ɛ/	/ɛ/	as in head	/hɛd/	_______	red	_______	/rɛd/
/æ/	/æ/	as in hat	/hæt/	_______	sat	_______	/sæt/
/ʊ/	/ʊ/	as in hood	/hʊd/	_______	good	_______	/gʊd/
/ɔ/	/ɔ/	as in haul	/hɔl/	_______	ball	_______	/bɔl/
/ʌ/	/ʌ/	as in hut	/hʌt/	_______	rut	_______	/rʌt/
/ə/	/ə/	as in above	/ə'bʌv/	_______	a rut	_______	/ə'rʌt/
/ɝ/	/ɝ/	as in heard	/hɝd/	_______	word	_______	/wɝd/
/ɚ/	/ɚ/	as in header	/hɛdɚ/	_______	deader	_______	/dɛdɚ/
/j͜u/	/j͜u/	as in hue	/hj͜u/	_______	cue	_______	/kj͜u/
/ɔ͜ɪ/	/ɔ͜ɪ/	as in hoist	/hɔ͜ɪst/	_______	moist	_______	/mɔ͜ɪst/
/a͜ʊ/	/a͜ʊ/	as in how	/ha͜ʊ/	_______	cow	_______	/ka͜ʊ/
/a͜ɪ/	/a͜ɪ/	as in high	/ha͜ɪ/	_______	buy	_______	/ba͜ɪ/

Audio-Activity 1.3. New Symbols for the Vowels and Diphthongs (CD 1, Track 3)

For this Audio-Activity, you will hear each new vowel sound followed by a key word. Transcribe *only* the new symbol for each vowel. You will probably have to listen to this activity several times while you look at the answers. Then cover the answers and work slowly until your performance is near perfect on these 26 items.

		Answers	
1. _______	2. _______	/ɪ/	/ɛ/
3. _______	4. _______	/æ/	/ʊ/
5. _______	6. _______	/ɔ/	/ʌ/
7. _______	8. _______	/ə/	/ɝ/
9. _______	10. _______	/ɚ/	/j͜u/
11. _______	12. _______	/ɔ͜ɪ/	/a͜ʊ/
13. _______	14. _______	/a͜ɪ/	/a͜ʊ/
15. _______	16. _______	/ɪ/	/ʊ/
17. _______	18. _______	/ɚ/	/ɝ/
19. _______	20. _______	/ɔ͜ɪ/	/a͜ɪ/
21. _______	22. _______	/ʌ/	/j͜u/
23. _______	24. _______	/ə/	/ɛ/
25. _______	26. _______	/æ/	/ɔ/

The Consonant Symbols

Symbol Printed Form	Symbol Written Form						
/ŋ/	/ŋ/	as in sing	/sɪŋ/	_______	ring	_______	/rɪŋ/
/ʃ/	/ʃ/	as in shin	/ʃɪn/	_______	ship	_______	/ʃɪp/
/ʒ/	/ʒ/	as in treasure	/trɛʒɚ/	_______	measure	_______	/mɛʒɚ/
/tʃ/	/tʃ/	as in chin	/tʃɪn/	_______	chip	_______	/tʃɪp/
/dʒ/	/dʒ/	as in gin	/dʒɪn/	_______	gyp	_______	/dʒɪp/
/θ/	/θ/	as in thin	/θɪn/	_______	thick	_______	/θɪk/
/ð/	/ð/	as in then	/ðɛn/	_______	them	_______	/ðɛm/

Audio-Activity 1.4. New Symbols for the Consonants (CD 1, Track 4)

For this activity, we will use the same procedure that we used for learning the new vowel and diphthong symbols. First, review the new consonant symbols. Then continue with the 14 sounds in this list. As before, we will use the vowel /ɪ/ to make these sounds clearer, even though the vowel in the key word may be different. Transcribe only the symbol for the new consonant. Check your answers after you have mastered these symbols.

		Answers	
1. _______	2. _______	/ŋ/	/ʃ/
3. _______	4. _______	/ʒ/	/tʃ/
5. _______	6. _______	/dʒ/	/θ/
7. _______	8. _______	/ð/	/dʒ/
9. _______	10. _______	/ʒ/	/ŋ/
11. _______	12. _______	/ð/	/tʃ/
13. _______	14. _______	/θ/	/ʃ/

Obviously, nothing is as simple as it first appears. Therefore, expect to find other symbols and variations to this basic set of symbols as you progress in your study. At this point, you should have some notion of the task awaiting you and a strategy for making each sound-symbol association. If the task seems difficult, remember that you already have had some practice using 22 of the symbols of the IPA Alphabet.

Developing Metaphonological Awareness

One ability you need to develop as a budding transcriber is the facility to deal with speech as a complex system isolated from meaning. Transcribers focus on the *form* of speech, not its *content* or *function*. In so doing, speech sounds take on a reality of their own; they are no longer secondary to the message but supersede the message. Speech becomes an end unto itself as emphasis is placed solely on the manner and production of sounds.

In the real world we place much less emphasis on the form of speech because meaning is central to communication. When a slip-of-the-tongue occurs, however, our attention is frequently drawn to the form of speech. Such attention to form is known as *metaphonological awareness*, and for many of us it is a skill that must be developed more fully before we become expert transcribers.

Meta- is a prefix that means transcending. When we are conscious of speech by trying to analyze, explain, or transcribe it, we enter the realm of *metaphonology*. Sounds, symbols, syllables, and stresses are the raw material of metaphonology. Whenever we make a pun ("Kansas is Oz-some") or rhyme words in a poem ("Hickory dickory dock, the mouse ran up the clock"), we use metaphonological abilities.

Although we are born with considerable skill in acquiring sounds, syllables, and stresses, we do not become metaphonologically aware until much later in life, and all of us have to make a conscious effort to develop this cognitive ability as we study to become transcribers of speech. The exercises that follow will help you to understand metaphonological awareness and start you on the road to developing the needed skills.

Exercise 1.4. How Many Sounds?

In this exercise, determine how many sounds, not necessarily letters, make up each word and write the number in the corresponding space. Cover the answers, then check your decisions.

		Number of Sounds	Answers
Example:	phonetics	___	8
	dog	___	3
	scab	___	4
	telegraph	___	8
	tugboat	___	6
	chrome	___	4
	monologue	___	7
	gymnasium	___	9

Exercise 1.5. Differentiating Consonants and Vowels

Now that you know how to determine the number of sounds in words, you can now differentiate those sounds in *vowels* and *consonants*. For producing vowel sounds, the vocal tract is open; when producing the consonants, there is usually a closure. As before, cover the answers until you have finished.

		Number of Consonants	Number of Vowels	Answers	
Example:	phonetics	___	___	5	2
	dog	___	___	2	1
	scab	___	___	3	1
	telegraph	___	___	5	3
	tugboat	___	___	4	2
	chrome	___	___	3	1
	monologue	___	___	4	3
	gymnasium	___	___	5	4

Exercise 1.6. How Many Syllables?

As you pronounce these words, determine the number of *syllables* (pulses or beats) that each has. A good technique is to tap on something as you say each word, letting the number of taps represent each syllable. Cover the answers as you write your answer in the space provided and then check it.

	Number of Syllables		Answers
Example:	phonetics	___	3
	simplification	___	5
	committed	___	3
	liquidate	___	3
	electrician	___	4
	nephew	___	2
	psychology	___	4
	geometrical	___	5
	rehabilitation	___	6

Exercise 1.7. Selecting the Prominent or Stressed Syllable

Using the same words as in the previous exercise, try to determine which syllable is prominent (stressed) and write the number corresponding to that syllable in the space provided. For example, the stressed syllable in *alphabet* is syllable 1—*AL-pha-bet*. The stressed syllable is higher in pitch and slightly louder than the other syllables in the word. Again, cover the answers while you work, and then check your work against the answers.

	Stressed Syllable		Answers
Example:	phonetics	___	2
	simplification	___	4
	committed	___	2
	liquidate	___	1
	electrician	___	3
	nephew	___	1
	psychology	___	2
	geometrical	___	3
	rehabilitation	___	5

Exercise 1.8. Rhyming Words

Another way to develop metaphonological skills is by rhyming words. Begin to work on this ability by writing two words that rhyme with each of these one syllable words.

Example:	my	by sky
	your	____________
	meet	____________
	ask	____________
	boat	____________
	head	____________
	should	____________
	fat	____________
	king	____________
	sound	____________
	pipe	____________

CONSONANT CHART FOR AMERICAN ENGLISH

- as used in this text -

	Bilabial	Labiodental	Dental	Alveolar	Palatal	Velar	Glottal
Stop	p b			t d		k g	
Nasal	m			n		ŋ	
Fricative		f v	θ ð	s z	ʃ ʒ		h
Lateral				l			
Affricate					tʃ dʒ		
Approximant	w			r	j	(w)	

Note: Where symbols appear in pairs, the first is voiceless, the second voiced.

VOWELS & DIPHTHONGS FOR AMERICAN ENGLISH

VOWELS

	Front	Central	Back
High	i		u
Lower High	ɪ		ʊ
Mid	e	ʌ ə ɝ ɚ	o
Lower Mid	ɛ		ɔ
Higher Low	æ		ɒ
Low	a		ɑ

DIPHTHONGS

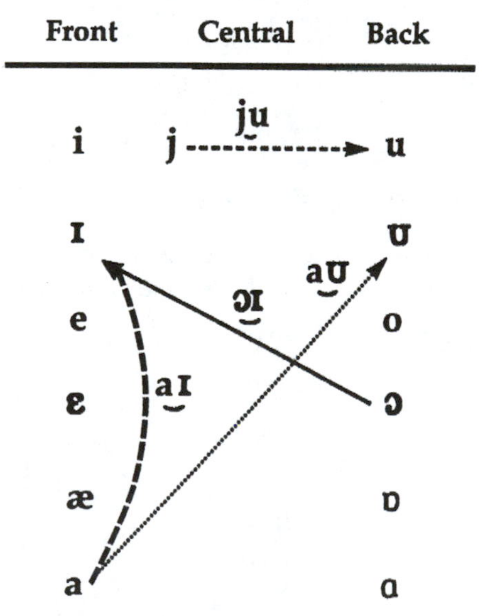

Note: Where symbols appear in pairs, the first is stressed, the second unstressed.

Figure 1-1
The phonetic alphabet, based on the International Phonetic Association alphabet, revised to 1996.

Using the Flash Cards

A complete set of phonetic flash cards is provided with this book. Keep them with you so that you can learn to make the sound-symbol associations as quickly and easily as possible. Here are some suggested activities for using the cards.

1. Go through the deck slowly by looking at the symbol and saying the corresponding sound. Check your pronunciation by looking at the key words on the other side of the card.
2. Gradually increase your speed and accuracy. Randomize the cards each time you go through the deck.
3. Go through the cards as quickly as you can. If you hesitate on any card, set it aside for additional drill.
4. Sort the vowels, diphthongs, and consonants into three piles. Go through each by sounding out the symbol on each card. Increase your speed. Strive for automaticity in responding to the cards. The sound-symbol association must be fast, accurate, and automatic. Speed is essential in real-time phonetic transcription.
5. Arrange the flash cards for the consonants into the vertical and horizontal classes as in the consonant chart in Figure 1-1, and learn to recognize the sounds within each class.
6. Arrange the flash cards for the vowels and diphthongs as in the vowel and diphthong diagram in Figure 1-1 and say each one in order: first top to bottom, then bottom to top; front to back, then back to front. Increase your speed as you drill.
7. Learn any special names for sounds, such as *ash* for /æ/ and *esh* for /ʃ/.
8. Learn the classical phonetic description for each sound, such as "Voiceless (Lingua-) Velar Stop" for /k/.
9. Working with a friend, preferably someone who is studying phonetics with you, go through activities 1 to 8 in this series.
10. Study every day. Make sure that you are not practicing the wrong sound-symbol associations.

Audio-Activity 1.5. Using the Flash Cards for the Standard IPA Symbols (CD 1, Track 5)

Prepare the flash cards for use and stack them in numerical order, that is, by the number found in the upper left-hand corner of each card. When you are ready, listen for each sound *and* for a key word containing that sound. First *say* the sound aloud, then repeat the key word out loud. Finally, transcribe *only* the sound in the space provided. There are 42 items. This time we will add the vowel /ʌ/ to the consonants to make them easier to hear. Cover the answers as you work and then check your work against the answers.

		Answers	
1. _______	2. _______	/p/	/b/
3. _______	4. _______	/t/	/d/
5. _______	6. _______	/k/	/g/
7. _______	8. _______	/f/	/v/
9. _______	10. _______	/θ/	/ð/
11. _______	12. _______	/s/	/z/
13. _______	14. _______	/ʃ/	/ʒ/
15. _______	16. _______	/h/	/tʃ/
17. _______	18. _______	/dʒ/	/m/
19. _______	20. _______	/n/	/ŋ/

21. _______	22. _______	/j/	/w/
23. _______	24. _______	/r/	/l/
25. _______	26. _______	/i/	/ɪ/
27. _______	28. _______	/e/	/ɛ/
29. _______	30. _______	/æ/	/ʌ/
31. _______	32. _______	/ə/	/ɝ/
33. _______	34. _______	/ɚ/	/u/
35. _______	36. _______	/ʊ/	/o/
37. _______	38. _______	/ɔ/	/ɑ/
39. _______	40. _______	/a͜ɪ/	/a͜ʊ/
41. _______	42. _______	/ɔ͜ɪ/	/j͜u/

The rest of the flash cards contain sounds that will be introduced later.

Audio-Activity 1.6. A Speed Drill with the Flash Cards: Consonants (CD 1, Track 6)

Take flash cards 1 to 24, for the consonants, and arrange them in numerical order in front of you. You will hear a sound and keyword. As before, we will use the vowel /ʌ/ with each consonant to make it more intelligible, although the vowel in the keyword may be different. Locate the symbol from the array of flash cards in front of you and form a pile of the cards as used. Speed is desired for this activity. There is nothing to transcribe. Continue with this activity until you reach mastery. The answers are provided for checking your work.

Answers

1. /v/ 2. /d/ 3. /h/ 4. /ʃ/ 5. /n/ 6. /θ/ 7. /j/ 8. /p/ 9. /tʃ/ 10. /f/ 11. /dʒ/
12. /w/ 13. /z/ 14. /r/ 15. /b/ 16. /l/ 17. /ð/ 18. /k/ 19. /m/ 20. /t/ 21. /ʒ/
22. /s/ 23. /ŋ/ 24. /g/

Audio-Activity 1.7. A Speed Drill with the Flash Cards: Vowels and Diphthongs (CD 1, Track 7)

Now use flash cards 25 to 42, for the vowels and diphthongs. Arrange the cards in front of you as you did for Audio-Activity 1.6. Work for speed as you locate a card and stack it on the previous one. There is nothing to transcribe; you are working with this set of flashcards. Answers are provided so that you can check your accuracy. There are 18 items.

Answers

1. /ɝ/ 2. /ʌ/ 3. /e/ 4. /ɔ͜ɪ/ 5. /u/ 6. /o/ 7. /ɑ/ 8. /j͜u/ 9. /ɛ/ 10. /ɪ/ 11. /ʊ/
12. /a͜ɪ/ 13. /i/ 14. /ɔ/ 15. /ɚ/ 16. /ə/ 17. /æ/ 18. /a͜ʊ/

Audio-Activity 1.8. Using the Flash Cards for the New Consonant Symbols (CD 1, Track 8)

This activity is designed to provide additional work with the new consonant symbols. Locate flash cards 6, 9, 10, 13, 14, 16, 17, 20, and 21, and then arrange them within view in front of you. Listen to the sound and key word. Then repeat both the sound and the key word as you look at each card. There is nothing to transcribe.

Audio-Activity 1.9. Using the Flash Cards for the Vowels and Diphthongs (CD 1, Track 9)

Organize the flash cards in order from 25 to 42. Listen to the sound and key word. Then repeat each sound and key word as you look at its flash card. There is nothing to transcribe.

Audio-Activity 1.10. Practice in Using Appendix A (CD 1, Track 10)

Open your workbook to Appendix A, where you will see the Printed and Handwritten Symbols. Review the handwritten symbols in the third column. Now listen to each sound and its corresponding key word as you look at Appendix A. When you have automatic control of each symbol, replay CD 1, Track 10, and write the symbols in the space provided. When you have finished, confirm your transcriptions with the versions in Appendix A. There are 46 items to transcribe. As usual, the consonants are pronounced in isolation with the vowel /ʌ/.

Using *Applied Phonetics: The Sounds of American English*

The following sections of this text contain Learning Activities for which the text, *Applied Phonetics: The Sounds of American English*, is used. These Learning Activities will acquaint you with the sounds that you will be transcribing—how they are described by phoneticians, their common spellings, and other characteristics important to their specification. The Learning Activities should be considered as relevant to learning the sounds as the Transcription Exercises.

The data on each of the speech sounds included in the text are organized similarly for each sound for easy reference. Place special emphasis on the beginning overview chapters and on the introductory description for each of the sounds of American English.

SECTION 2

Consonants: /p, b, t, d, k, g, m, n, ŋ, l, r/
Vowels: /ɪ, ɛ, æ, ə, ɚ, o/

■ Learning Activities to Introduce the Sounds in Section 2

Before learning to transcribe the sounds in this section, you should become familiar with them as speech sounds, so as to make talking about and transcribing them easier. These Learning Activities are designed to acquaint you with the sounds and to instruct you in the use of the companion text to this workbook, *Applied Phonetics: The Sounds of American English (AP)*; Part II contains detailed information on each of the speech sounds of American English. Follow the instructions carefully as you work through the Learning Activities.

Learning Activity 2.1. The Stop Consonants: /p, b, t, d, k, g/

Turn to Chapter 5 in *Applied Phonetics: The Sounds of American English (AP)* and read the Introduction to the Stop Consonants. Notice that the information for each sound is organized in the same way and with the most general information placed first. Then complete the following Learning Activities using the data from Chapter 5 in *AP* as directed.

1. Define the term *stop*: ______________________________
2. List the three voiceless stops: ______________________________
3. List the three voiced stops: ______________________________
4. What sound is the voiceless bilabial stop? ______________________________
5. What sound is the voiced alveolar stop? ______________________________
6. What sound is the voiced velar stop? ______________________________
7. What sound is the voiceless alveolar stop? ______________________________
8. For what stops is tongue position irrelevant? ______________________________
9. For what stops is the tongue back raised? ______________________________
10. For what stops is the tongue front raised? ______________________________
11. Which stops have closure of the passageway into the nose? ______________________________
12. Among non-native speakers of American English, what might be a primary source of production difficulty for the stop consonants? ______________________________

Learning Activity 2.2. True/False Questions

Answer the following questions by circling T for true or F for false.

T F 1. All stops require a complete closure at some point within the vocal tract.

T F 2. As a group, the stops have consistent spellings in English.

T F 3. As a group, the stops appear early in the speech of children acquiring English as their native language

T F 4. Some scholars consider the nasal phonemes to be stops.

T F 5. Another term used to refer to the stops is *explosives*.

Learning Activity 2.3. The Nasal Consonants: /m, n, ŋ/

Study the material in Chapter 8 in *AP* on the nasal consonants. As before, read the Introduction. Then use the data under each sound to complete this Learning Activity.

1. The nasals are produced differently from all of the other sounds in English. What is the primary difference? ______
2. What nasal consonant is most like the stop /k/? ______
3. What nasal consonant is most like the stop /b/? ______
4. What nasal consonant is most like the stop /t/? ______
5. What is the difference between the nasals and the voiced stops in terms of:

   voicing? ______

   velopharyngeal closure? ______

   tongue position? ______
6. What nasal consonant is the voiced alveolar nasal? ______
7. What nasal consonant is bilabial? ______
8. What nasal consonant is the voiced velar nasal? ______
9. Which of the nasals is not found in initial word position in English? ______
10. What nasal is most likely to need remediation in the speech of non-native speakers of American English? ______

Learning Activity 2.4. The Consonants: /l, r/

Chapter 9 (pp. 187–215) in *AP* contains information on /r/ and /l/ (pp. 202–215). Read the introductory material on these sounds, survey the data on each, and then complete this Learning Activity.

1. /l/ and /r/ are often grouped together and called: ______
2. Which of these sounds is also known as the lateral? ______
3. Phoneticians call /r/ the voiced ______ glide or approximant.
4. Dewey (1971) presents 11 different spellings for /r/. How many spellings does he report for /l/? ______

   ______

5. Which of these two sounds is made with slight lip-rounding? ______
6. Are /l/ and /r/ difficult sounds for many non-native speakers of American English? ______
7. /l/ is most like what stop consonant? ______
8. /l/ is most like what nasal consonant? ______

Learning Activity 2.5. The Vowels: /ɪ, ɛ, æ, ə, ɚ, o/

Look up each of these six vowels in *AP*. You will use Chapters 10 (pp. 222, 233, 239), 11 (pp. 252, 263), and 12 (pp. 282). Then fill in the blanks in the Learning Activity that follows.

1. Of these six vowels, which are front vowels? ______
2. Of these vowels, which one is a back vowel? ______
3. Name the one vowel in this series that is *tense*. ______
4. For which sound does Dewey (1971) report 33 different spellings? ______
5. Which vowel is known as the *schwa*? ______
6. Which two vowels in this set may function as neutral (or reduced) vowels in American English? ______
7. Which two vowels do not regularly end words in English?______
8. Which of these sounds is questionable in word final position? ______
9. Which vowel in this list do phoneticians frequently treat as a diphthong? ______
10. Which vowel is the *mid-central, r-colored, lax vowel*? ______

Guidelines for Transcribers

Remember that it is not necessary to use slashes or brackets on workbook transcriptions.

Phonetic transcribers should make each symbol as carefully and as neatly as possible. If your handwriting is highly stylized or flowery, you will have to adjust so that your work looks like this:

gig ɡɪɡ
met mɛt
bang bæŋ
bone bon

Some Common Transcription Errors: Five Warnings

1. **Do not over-pronounce**. In transcribing words, beginners sometimes pronounce very slowly and carefully, distorting the sounds, particularly the vowels. For example, the word *bedded* is correctly transcribed as /ˈbɛdəd/ with a reduced vowel (schwa) in the second syllable. Beginning transcribers, pronouncing each syllable with too much precision, are tempted to mistranscribe the reduced vowel by using /ɛ/.
2. **Do not capitalize symbols in names**. The name Rob is transcribed just like the verb rob: /ˈrɑb/. IPA symbols do not come in upper and lower case. When a capital letter is used as a phonetic symbol, it represents a different sound and must always represent that sound with the capitalized symbol. For example, the symbol /r/ stands for one sound and /R/ represents another.
3. **Silent letters in words are not transcribed**. Some words in English contain letters that are not pronounced. Perhaps they were spoken at one time in history, but have now become silent. Which sounds are not pronounced in *lamb, knee, sigh*, and *make*? Although it is easy to see that *make* ends with a

silent *e*, you may be surprised to learn that *packed* contains six letters, but its transcription requires only four phonetic symbols: /ˈpækt/.

4. **No double letters are permitted within words**. Although letters standing for consonants are often doubled in English spelling, the sounds that they stand for are not doubled. Thus *begged* has only one /g/ sound: /ˈbɛgd/. Later we will see that a sound used to terminate one word and release the next, such as in *weighed down*, may be transcribed so as to preserve word boundaries by doubling the two /d/s, but with a space between.

5. **Marks of punctuation are not transcribed**. No commas, periods, apostrophes, or other marks of punctuation are used in transcribing. In writing, an apostrophe may represent a reduced vowel, as in *Bess's* (/ˈbɛsəz/).

Learning to Transcribe These Sounds: Consonants: /p, b, t, d, k, g, m, n, ŋ, l, r/ Vowels: /ɪ, ɛ, æ, ə, ɚ, o/

Introduction

The first sounds that you will learn to transcribe will be two sets of consonants—the stops and the nasals—and a few vowels. These sounds are particularly easy for students to learn and, therefore, provide a good starting point for the study of phonetic transcription. Ten of the 11 consonant symbols that mark the beginning of our study are familiar because they are identical in form and pronunciation to 10 letters in the English alphabet. It should be noted, however, that the phonetic symbol /g/ stands only for the stop sound corresponding to the alphabet letter *g* and represents this sound in *get, big*, and *agree*. This is not the sound of *g* in *gem, age*, or *plagiarize*, which will be represented by a different symbol to be practiced later. In addition to standing for the sound normally signaled by the letter *k*, the symbol /k/ will also stand for the same sound when written in English with a *c* (the so-called hard *c*, as in *cat*).

The four vowels that are used in the first transcription exercises are symbolized by /ɪ/, /ɛ/, /æ/, and /o/. Only /o/ is a letter of the alphabet. Therefore, special caution is needed in making the three new symbols. Do not forget to cap the /ɪ/, and pay particular attention to the instructions for making the /æ/ in Transcription Exercise 2.3.

Transcription Exercises

Transcription Exercise 2.1. The Vowel Sound /ɪ/

Transcribe these words containing the /ɪ/ sound, as in *bit*.

bit ____________	tip ____________
kit ____________	mitt ____________
bib ____________	pick ____________
dig ____________	big ____________

Transcription Exercise 2.2. The Vowel /ɛ/

Transcribe these words containing the /ɛ/ sound, as in *bet*.

bet ____________	beg ____________
net ____________	let ____________
bed ____________	Ben ____________
get ____________	met ____________

Transcription Exercise 2.3. The Vowel /æ/

Transcribe these words containing the /æ/ sound, as in *bat*.
Handy hint: To make the symbol /æ/, three steps are necessary:

1. Beginning at the top left of the letter, trace the symbol /ɔ/: ɔ ɔ
2. Without lifting the pencil, close the loop, /ə/: ə ə
3. Without lifting the pencil, add the handwritten letter *e*, /e/: æ æ

1. ɔ   2. ə   3. æ

Note: The symbols /ɔ/ and /ə/ are two additional IPA alphabet symbols that will be studied later.

bat________	gag________
gnat________	dam________
pan________	pal________
nag________	Matt________

Transcription Exercise 2.4. The Vowel /o/

Transcribe these words containing the /o/ sound, as in *boat*. There is no /ow/ in IPA transcription.

boat________	low________
loan________	don't________
nope________	poke________
goat________	tow________

Audio-Activity 2.1. A Decision-Making Activity (CD 1, Track 11)

This is a discrimination exercise for the vowels /ɪ/ as in *bit*, /ɛ/ as in *bet*, /æ/ as in *bat*, and /o/ as in *boat*. Review flash cards 26, 28, 29, and 36. Then listen to each of these words. If a given word has one of these four vowels, write the symbol for the vowel in the space provided. If the word does *not* have one of them, write "No." Each of these 16 words will be pronounced once. The words for 12 through 15 have two syllables and require two answers each. Cover the answers as you work, then check your work against the answers.

		Answers	
1. ______	2. ______	/ɪ/	No
3. ______	4. ______	/o/	No
5. ______	6. ______	No	/ɪ/
7. ______	8. ______	/ɛ/	/æ/
9. ______	10. ______	No	No
11. ______	12. ______	No	/æ/, No
13. ______	14. ______	No, No	No, /æ/
15. ______	16. ______	/ɛ/, No	/o/

Audio-Activity 2.2. The Vowel /ɪ/ *(CD 1, Track 12)*

Transcribe these six words that contain the /ɪ/ vowel.

		Answers	
1. ______	2. ______	ˈbɪt	ˈkɪk
3. ______	4. ______	ˈmɪnt	ˈpɪk
5. ______	6. ______	ˈtɪp	ˈtɪkt

Audio-Activity 2.3. The Vowel /ɛ/ (CD 1, Track 13)

Transcribe these six words that contain the /ɛ/ vowel.

1. ________	2. ________
3. ________	4. ________
5. ________	6. ________

Answers

ˈmɛn	ˈdɛt
ˈdɛk	ˈnɛd
ˈpɛt	ˈtɛd

Audio-Activity 2.4. The Vowel /æ/ (CD 1, Track 14)

Transcribe these six words that contain the /æ/ vowel.

1. ________	2. ________
3. ________	4. ________
5. ________	6. ________

Answers

ˈkæt	ˈtæk
ˈmæd	ˈtæn
ˈtæp	ˈtæb

Audio-Activity 2.5. The Vowel /o/ (CD 1, Track 15)

Transcribe these six words that contain the /o/ vowel.

1. ________	2. ________
3. ________	4. ________
5. ________	6. ________

Answers

ˈkod	ˈton
ˈnon	ˈkop
ˈmon	ˈbot

Transcription Exercise 2.5. Review

Each of the following words can be transcribed with three of the set of symbols introduced for study in this section. *Remember: You cannot use any phonetic symbols that have not been presented in this section of the workbook.* Even if the vowel in a word seems different, the way you normally say it, from any of the four vowels you are learning to use, transcribe the word with the vowel most likely to be used by many other speakers. You might want to put an asterisk (*) by the word so that you can return to it later. For example, in some dialects *keg* is pronounced with a vowel other than /ɪ ɛ, æ, o/.

You may check your transcriptions for the 20 items in the left-hand column by looking in Appendix B of this workbook: Selected Answers to Some Transcription Exercises.

pit ____________________	comb ____________________
cone ____________________	gnat ____________________
gag ____________________	tact ____________________
dough ____________________	did ____________________
dope ____________________	peck ____________________
cab ____________________	moan ____________________
debt ____________________	Mack ____________________
knack ____________________	cat ____________________
owe ____________________	keg ____________________
gap ____________________	node ____________________

bad ________	tip ________
mow ________	back ________
kin ________	towed ________
dead ________	ma'am ________
act ________	neck ________
known ________	know ________
man ________	bag ________
bid ________	mope ________
net ________	peg ________
lap ________	knit ________

Audio-Activity 2.6. Review of the Vowels /ɪ/, /æ/, /ɛ/, and /o/ (CD 1, Track 16)

Transcribe these six words (with the answers covered). Then check you work.

		Answers	
1. ________	2. ________	ˈpæŋ	ˈmæm
3. ________	4. ________	ˈnɪt	ˈnɛk
5. ________	6. ________	ˈnod	ˈdɛd

Audio-Activity 2.7. Transcribing Nonsense Words (CD 1, Track 17)

Here are six nonsense items for further practice on these vowels.

		Answers	
1. ________	2. ________	ˈnɪd	ˈkæk
3. ________	4. ________	ˈmom	ˈmɪb
5. ________	6. ________	ˈgɛd	ˈgop

Transcription Exercise 2.6. Introducing /ŋ/ as in ink

Transcribe these words containing the /ŋ/ sound. There are two things to remember that will make your transcription easier. First, in spelling, /ŋ/ stands for the sound often spelled *ng* as in *sang*. Second, it also stands for the sound spelled *n* when it occurs before /k/ or /g/. For example, *bank* is not the word *ban* followed by a /k/; it is the word *bang* followed by a /k/: /ˈbæŋk/. When you have finished transcribing these words, check your answers in Appendix B of this workbook.

Warning: For the vowel sounds in these words, use only the four vowel symbols that have been introduced so far in this section, even if your dialect differs.

king ________	gang ________
ink ________	ping ________
tank ________	bank ________
pink ________	ding ________
tang ________	bang ________

Transcription Exercise 2.7. Transcribing Words with /l/ and /r/

In addition to the symbols used in previous Transcription Exercises, you will be adding /l/ as in *link* and /r/ as in *rink*. These symbols usually represent the sounds that the letters *l* and *r* represent in spelling. Although there are complications associated with these sounds, we will begin with simple transcriptions, leaving the transcription problems for later. Check your work by using Appendix B of this workbook.

land ____________________	plaque ____________________
chrome ____________________	dread ____________________
rib ____________________	cling ____________________
roan ____________________	rink ____________________
wreck ____________________	load ____________________
rill ____________________	pole ____________________
bring ____________________	crib ____________________
blown ____________________	drag ____________________

Audio-Activity 2.8. Listening for /l/ *and* /r/ *(CD 1, Track 18)*

Before doing this activity, you should review flash cards 23 for /r/ and 24 for /l/. Transcribe these six words. Then check your answers against those given.

1. ________ 2. ________
3. ________ 4. ________
5. ________ 6. ________

Answers

ˈkrom	ˈblæbd
ˈtrɛd	ˈtrɪkt
ˈrol	ˈlækt

Audio-Activity 2.9. Nonsense Words with /l/ *or* /r/ *(CD 1, Track 19)*

Transcribe each of these six nonsense items, which contain either /l/ or /r/ as well as other sounds that you have been practicing. As always, cover the answers until you are ready to check your work.

1. ________ 2. ________
3. ________ 4. ________
5. ________ 6. ________

Answers

ˈglɪmp	ˈblop
ˈdræk	ˈplɛl
ˈtrom	ˈkræŋ

The Pitch Test, Marking Primary Stress, and Vowel Reduction with /ə/

In the transcriptions so far, the words have usually been one syllable long. There are several complications for transcribing words of more than one syllable, but only two need to be discussed here. First, in such words one syllable is usually pronounced with greater stress (or emphasis), often reflected as a jump upward in pitch on that syllable (Section 7 has a more complete description of American English stress). For example, in the word *cola*, the first syllable receives the pitch jump whereas the other syllable is unstressed (or weaker) and falls in pitch: *COla*. In the word *ago*, the second syllable has the pitch jump: *aGO*. So, one complication is caused by the need to mark levels of stress.

One way to determine where the stress occurs in words is to apply the pitch test. Pronounce the word naturally to determine which syllable receives the jump in pitch. Try the pitch test on *cola* and *ago* by making the pitch of your voice conform to the contour of each of these diagrams:

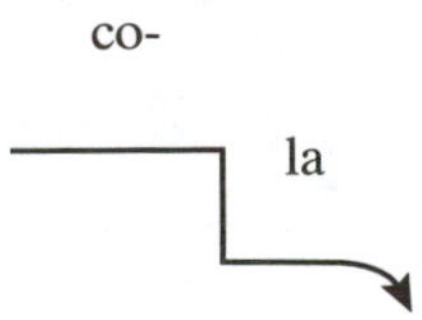

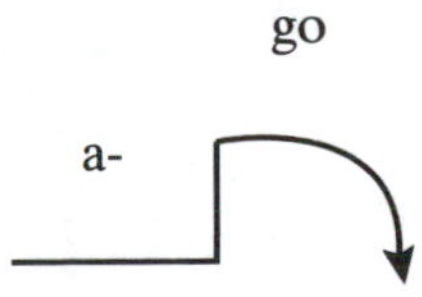

Note: The last syllable in these words ends with a fall in pitch, denoted by the arrow. Even in words that require a pitch jump on the last syllable, as in *ago*, there is still a final fall in pitch. This fall in pitch serves to tell our listener that the word has ended.

The way that primary stress is marked varies from dictionary to dictionary and from one transcription system to another (for more information, see Section 13). The IPA has opted for a raised vertical mark placed *before* the stressed syllable: /ˈ/. Thus, the transcription of *cola* is /ˈkolə/ and of *ago* is /əˈgo/.

A second complication is caused by the process of vowel reduction, which is very important in American English. The vowel in the unstressed syllables of *cola* and *ago* is reduced. There is a special symbol for the sound of this reduced vowel and it is called the *schwa*: /ə/. It only occurs in unstressed syllables, never in syllables that receive the pitch jump.

Warning: The articles *the* and *a* are usually pronounced with the reduced schwa vowel. Notice that in *the map* and *a map*, the pitch jump occurs on *map*.

Transcription Exercise 2.8. Practice with the Pitch Test, Marking Primary Stress, and Vowel Reduction with /ə/

a. Apply the pitch test to these four words by drawing a pitch contour like those already shown for *cola* and *ago*.

Tampa abode

talcum lapel

b. Now transcribe this set of words, putting a primary stress mark before the stressed syllable or marking it as your instructor tells you. Use the schwa (/ə/) to represent the reduced vowel of the unstressed syllable. You may check your transcription of the first three items in each column in Appendix B of this workbook.

Words Stressed on the First Syllable	**Words Stressed on the Second Syllable**
Tampa________	abode________
talcum________	amid ________
Alan________	abet________
camel________	akin ________
Anna________	alone________
opal________	lapel ________
okra________	inept ________

Audio-Activity 2.10. Using the Reduced Vowel /ə/ (CD 1, Track 20)

Examine flash card 31. Then use the schwa to represent the reduced vowels in the words you hear. Transcribe these words, marking the stressed syllable in each word. There are six items.

1. ________ 2. ________
3. ________ 4. ________
5. ________ 6. ________

Answers

ˈɛlən	əˈton
kəˈmɪt	əˈkɪn
ˈokrə	əˈdæpt

Vowel Reduction with /ɪ/

There are two neutral or reduced vowels in American English. One of these is the schwa, /ə/; the other is /ɪ/. Notice the word *mimic*. Use the pitch test to determine which syllable receives primary stress. Which syllable is unstressed? Most speakers of English pronounce the unstressed syllable with /ɪ/ and would say /'mɪmɪk/. Notice that the vowel in both the stressed and unstressed syllables is essentially the same. Therefore, /ɪ/ can function as a *stressed* and *unstressed* vowel, whereas the schwa (/ə/) can function only as an *unstressed* vowel.

Transcription Exercise 2.9. Reduced Vowels

Transcribe this set of words using whichever of the two reduced vowel symbols best represents *your* pronunciation of the unstressed vowels, /ɪ/ or /ə/. Variation between these two vowels often occurs from speaker to speaker and also in the speech of the same speaker, even on repetitions of the same word. Continue, as always, to mark primary stress with a short vertical line (') in front of and slightly above the stressed syllable.

Check your answers to the words in the right-hand column by turning to Appendix B of this workbook.

panda________________	cryptic________________
epic________________	coma________________
cambric________________	tannic________________
mimic________________	cobra________________
attack________________	Mona________________
panic________________	bandit________________
limit________________	cabin________________
packet________________	boa________________
peptic________________	adept________________
adapt________________	delta ________________

Audio-Activity 2.11. Listening for the Reduced Vowels /ə/ and /ɪ/ (CD 1, Track 21)

Transcribe these six words listening carefully to the reduced vowels. Try to transcribe the one that actually occurs.

		Answers	
1. ________	2. ________	'bɛltɪd	'bɛltəd
3. ________	4. ________	'kæbən	'krɪptɪk
5. ________	6. ________	'bændɪt	ə'tæk

Vowel Reduction with the Unstressed Schwar /ɚ/, as in bidder

There is a special reduced vowel that has many of the same features as /r/. In the word *bidder*, the last syllable is unstressed and therefore has this reduced r-colored vowel. It is usually transcribed as /ɚ/, and the word *bidder* is transcribed as /'bɪdɚ/. An alternate transcription, although not employed in this text, is to write the last syllable of this word as schwa + r (e.g., /ər/), so that *bidder* would be /'bɪdər/. When the schwa and /r/ do not occur within the same syllable, they may be transcribed as two distinct sounds as in the word *aroma* (see Transcription Exercise 2.10).

Note: In some dialects of American and British English the sound represented by /ɚ/ does not occur. These dialects have only schwa in any of the positions where /ɚ/ might be used, so that *bicker* would be pronounced /'bɪkə/ and *bickered* would be /'bɪkəd/ (see Transcription Exercise 4.9). Check your answers to the first six items in the left column in Appendix B.

Transcription Exercise 2.10. Practice Transcribing /ɚ/

odor ______	aroma ______
erode ______	amber ______
planner ______	cracker ______
glimmer ______	polar ______
broker ______	dimmer ______
peppered ______	grammar ______
limber ______	braggart ______

Audio-Activity 2.12. Listening for /ɚ/ (CD 1, Track 22)

Transcribe the words that you hear using /ə/ (the schwa) and /ɚ/ (the schwar) where appropriate. Listen carefully because different dialect pronunciations occur. There are six words. When you finish, check your transcriptions with ours.

1. ______	2. ______
3. ______	4. ______
5. ______	6. ______

Answers

'lɪmbə	'græmɚ
ə'romə	'odə
'pɛpəd	'krækɚ

Transcription Exercise 2.11. Transcribing Words with Past Tense Endings

Transcribing *-ed* to show past tense can be confusing because this ending can be pronounced three different ways and, therefore, has three different phonetic transcriptions. When a verb ends with any voiceless consonant except /t/, the spelling *-ed* is pronounced as the voiceless stop /t/, as in *mapped* (/'mæpt/) and *packed* (/'pækt/). If any voiced consonant except /d/ ends the word, the *-ed* ending is pronounced as the voiced stop /d/, as in *tabbed* (/'tæbd/) and *begged* (/bɛgd/). Finally, if the verb ends with a /t/ or /d/ as in *netted* and *padded*, the past tense ending is pronounced and therefore transcribed as a separate syllable containing a reduced vowel (either /ə/ or /ɪ/) and /d/, for example, /'nɛtəd/ and /'pædəd/.

a. Transcribe these past tense words with /d/.

crammed ______	pinned ______
crowed ______	nabbed ______
clanged ______	begged ______
bragged ______	blabbed ______

b. Transcribe these past tense words with /t/.

camped ______	linked ______
groped ______	cracked ______
tricked ______	tripped ______
clapped ______	cranked ______

c. Transcribe these past tense words with /əd/.

kidded ______	dreaded ______
netted ______	padded ______

adapted_______________ added_______________

bloated_______________ matted _______________

d. Decide which of the three past tense endings to use in transcribing these words. Check your transcriptions to the first three words in each column in Appendix B.

batted _______________ knitted_______________

bagged_______________ mapped_______________

kidnaped_______________ lagged_______________

fretted _______________ licked_______________

gritted _______________ dipped_______________

Transcription Exercise 2.12. Review of Transcription Principles

Review all of the transcription principles discussed so far. Then transcribe the words, marking primary stress (even for words of only one syllable), and using the reduced vowels with /ə/ or /ɪ/ in the unstressed syllables. The first 10 items in the right column are transcribed in Appendix B.

Amanda _______________ editor_______________

omen_______________ dragon_______________

tipped _______________ moaned_______________

pink_______________ trimmed_______________

coped _______________ condone_______________

picker _______________ limited_______________

timid_______________ kidder_______________

combed_______________ owned_______________

trinket _______________ pecked_______________

cramped _______________ connected _______________

ribbon _______________ prank_______________

dabbed_______________ kept_______________

acted_______________ melted_______________

mammon_______________ redder_______________

a man _______________ credited_______________

a tone _______________ atoned_______________

Transcription Exercise 2.13. Optional Advanced Transcription

Some students may wish to transcribe words containing some of the sounds that will be introduced later. Perhaps you need to polish your skills quickly or want to test your ability to transcribe generally following your use of the flash cards. Here is a list of one- to three-syllable words containing some "new" sounds. The transcription principles that you have already learned still apply, however. Remember to mark primary stress appropriately.

twinkling_______________ splendor_______________

Mabel _______________ Hamilton _______________

combatant_______________ burgundy_______________

photograph _______________ satin_______________

rout ______________________	clarinet ______________________
freckle ______________________	spackle ______________________
botanical ______________________	crater ______________________
mitten ______________________	bitter ______________________
epsilon ______________________	initial ______________________
primitive ______________________	rattle ______________________

SECTION 3

Sound Variations in Phonetic Contexts, Registers, and Dialects
Consonants: [t̬, ɾ, ʔ]
Syllabics: [m̩, n̩, ŋ̩, l̩]
Vowel + /r/ Combination: /ɛr/

In reading the first three chapters in *Applied Phonetics: The Sounds of American English*, we quickly learn that human speech may vary along several important dimensions. The very nature of the English language determines how some sounds may be changed, even as a result of vowel reduction. As sounds occur with other sounds they may change. When we adapt our speech to a particular listener, we may use a manner of speech that is formal or informal. There are regional variations that are heard as we move from one part of the country to another. In this section, we will depart from learning the phonemes of American English to concentrate on some of the important ways that speech sounds are affected by these variables.

Intervocalic /t̬/

Notice that for many speakers of American English the sound that is spelled *t* or *tt* often is pronounced somewhat like a /d/ when it occurs between vowels and the vowel following does not carry stress. Hence the word *bitter* may sound like *bidder*. If these words sound different, they should be transcribed differently. Therefore, when orthographic *t* sounds like /d/, it should be transcribed with the diacritic for voicing, a small *v* (for voicing or partial voicing) placed under the /t/, or /t̬/. Using /d/ in such cases might lead to the conclusion that you had erred in transcription. In other words, a narrower approach to transcription is needed. Another reason that /d/ is not appropriate in such cases is that one would never pronounce *bitter* as *bidder* when making a very clear pronunciation such as in the example, "I said *bitter* not *bidder*."

Transcription Exercise 3.1. Contrasting /d/ and /t̬/

a. Transcribe these word pairs, using /d/ and /t̬/ as appropriate.

atom ______	Adam ______
debtor ______	deader ______
latter ______	ladder ______
bitter ______	bidder ______
matter ______	madder ______

b. Here are some words that you have transcribed in previous exercises. This time, use the intervocalic *t* as appropriate.

batted ______	fretted ______
gritted ______	netted ______
limited ______	credited ______
knitted ______	bloated ______

Audio-Activity 3.1. Listening for /t/, /d/, and /t̬/ (CD 1, Track 23)

Listen to these words and, for the consonant between the two vowels, write only the symbol for /t/, /d/, or voiced /t̬/ as necessary. There are six words. You do not have to transcribe the whole word. Cover the answers until you are ready to check your work.

		Answers	
1. ______	2. ______	/t/	/d/
3. ______	4. ______	/t̬/	/d/
5. ______	6. ______	/t̬/	/t/

The Alveolar Flap: An Alternate to /d/ and /t̬/

The alveolar flap (or tap) is transcribed like the /r/, except that the upper left serif is cut off /ɾ/. The /ɾ/ is an alternate for /t̬/ and can occur in many of the same environments. Because /t̬/ and /d/ are so similar, it is not surprising to find the alveolar flap as a variant form for both. In making this sound, which is phonemic in the Romance languages, the tongue literally flaps against the upper gum ridge. Acoustically, these sounds are very similar so that students often have difficulty differentiating among /bɛtɚ/, /bɛt̬ɚ/, and /bɛɾɚ/.

Transcription Exercise 3.2. The Alveolar Flap

Transcribe these words containing the intervocalic /t̬/ and /d/, but use their variant form, /ɾ/, the alveolar flap. Practice saying it.

letter ______	ladder ______
pattern ______	bitter ______
header ______	better ______
atom ______	debtor ______
betting ______	matting ______

Audio-Activity 3.2. Listening for /t̬/, /d/, or /ɾ/ (CD 1, Track 24)

Transcribe each word completely, using the alveolar flap instead of the voiced /t̬/, wherever it is pronounced. Otherwise, use /t/ or /d/. There are seven words to transcribe. Check your answers when finished.

		Answers	
1. ________	2. ________	ˈpæɾɚn	ˈhɛdɚ
3. ________	4. ________	ˈbotɪy	ˈmæɾɚ
5. ________	6. ________	ˈdɛtɚ	ˈdɛdɚ
7. ________		ˈdɛɾɚ	

Vowel Reduction: The Syllabic Consonants

In unstressed syllables the lateral /l/ and the nasal consonants /m/, /n/, and /ŋ/ may exhibit a kind of change involving vowel reduction, but different from the insertion of /ə/ or /ɪ/. Especially /l/ and /n/ show this kind of reduction. For example, most speakers of American English will not pronounce a vowel in the second syllable of the word *button*. Instead, they stop the airflow at the vocal cords with a glottal stop, /ʔ/ (see Transcription Exercise 3.5), and holding the position of the /t/, they switch the airflow to the nose, so that the /n/ is sounded without a vowel. Such an /n/ is called a syllabic consonant. The syllable consists primarily of the /n/ without a definite vowel being pronounced. The syllabic functions as *both* vowel and consonant in the syllable. The symbol for the syllabic /n/ is /n̩/, with a diacritic below it.

If the second syllable of *total* is pronounced without lifting the tongue tip from the alveolar ridge behind the upper teeth until the /l/ has been pronounced, a syllabic /l/ is produced. This time the airflow is momentarily stopped by a /t̬/, and is initiated again after the tongue is adjusted so that the /l̩/ sound can be produced, again without the presence of a true vowel. Syllabic /m̩/and /ŋ̩/ are also possible.

Sometimes a syllabic consonant is used by a speaker; at other times in the same word, a true vowel and consonant are produced. A syllabic consonant is more likely to occur when the articulators (the lips or tongue) do not move between the preceding sound and the lateral /l/ or nasal. In transcribing conversational speech, you will want to achieve competence in hearing the syllabics. The pointers given in "Preliminaries for Transcribing Syllabics" which follows, should help you gain this proficiency.

Preliminaries for Transcribing Syllabics

1. Syllabics are sounds that can function as the nucleus (center) of a syllable. All the vowels and five consonants—/m/, /n/, /ŋ/, /l/, and /r/—can function as syllabics. The vowels are syllabics in stressed and unstressed syllables, but *the consonants can only function as syllabics in unstressed (weaker) syllables*. Therefore, for syllabic /m/, /n/, /ŋ/, /l/, and /r/, a word of at least two syllables is required.
2. A diacritic, in this case a small vertical line placed *under* the symbol, is used to transform the symbols /m/, /n/, /ŋ/, and /l/ into representations for the syllabics: /m̩, n̩, ŋ̩, l̩/. Because /ɚ/ is the syllabic of /r/, no diacritic is used.
3. It is important to learn these syllabics. Speakers of American English use them as a preferred speech form.
4. These syllabics result from the loss of the preceding vowel. The vowel actually becomes part of the syllabic, so that

   /əm/ becomes /m̩/
   /ən/ becomes /n̩/
   /əŋ/ becomes /ŋ̩/
   /əl/ becomes /l̩/
   /ər/ becomes /ɚ/

5. Because the diacritic replaces the preceding vowel, no vowel will be found (a) before a syllabic or (b) in the same syllable with a syllabic.
6. With the exception of /l̩/ and /ɚ/, if a syllabic consonant is produced, it must bear a *homorganic relationship* with the preceding consonant in the same syllable. That is, they must be made with the same articulators as the sound before. In other words:

   /p and b/ will precede /m̩/ (bilabial articulation)

   /t, d, s, z/ will precede /n̩/ (alveolar articulation); /ʃ/ and /ʒ/ may precede n̩ (prepalatal articulation) /k and g/ will precede /ŋ̍/ (velar articulation)

   /ɚ/ and /l̩/ may be used after most consonants.
7. Syllabic /l̩/ or /ɚ/ preceded by /t/ will cause the /t/ to be pronounced as an intervocalic /t/ (or /t̬/). Compare *battle* and *batter*. Before syllabic /n̩/, /t/ will become a glottal stop /ʔ/, as in *batten*.
8. Many transcribers have adopted the convention of using the syllabic /ɚ/ with the vowel-plus-/r/ combination. That is, /ɑr/ becomes /ɑ͜ɚ/; /ir/ is /i͜ɚ/; /ɔr/ is transcribed /ɔ͜ɚ/; and /ɛr/ becomes /ɛ͜ɚ/. Because this convention violates the principle that the consonantal syllabics must form the nucleus of an unstressed syllable, we have decided against this common practice and use the traditional vowel + /r/ convention. For example, we use /ir/ not /i͜ɚ/. However, in narrower transcriptions, for productions of these vowel + /r/ combinations pronounced with a definite offglide, bordering on two syllables, we use vowel + /ɚ/ as when the word *fear* (/fir/) is pronounced with a definite offglide as /fi͜ɚ/. Learn to listen for these distinctions.

Transcription Exercise 3.3. Transcribing the Syllabic Consonants

The purpose of this exercise is to help you develop an awareness of vowel reduction through the use of syllabic consonants. Therefore, use the symbols for the syllabic consonants wherever possible. Remember that syllabic consonants are regularly preceded by consonants, not vowels. They will only occur in unstressed syllables, and when in a homorganic relationship with the preceding sound. (See item 6 in "Preliminaries for Transcribing Syllabics.") Don't forget to use the intervocalic [t̬] when it occurs before a syllabic /l̩/. (See item 7 in "Preliminaries.")

You may check your answers to the first five words in each column by turning to Appendix B. Some words are marked with an asterisk (*) indicating that no syllabic is transcribed. Do you know why? (See items 1 and 6 in "Preliminaries.")

*tilt ________________	redden ________________
middle ________________	wrinkle ________________
kettle ________________	ogle ________________
mitten ________________	brittle ________________
*kelp ________________	bitten ________________
pillar ________________	bidden ________________
molten ________________	tattle ________________
dimple ________________	panel ________________
*madam ________________	*colt ________________
madden ________________	trample ________________
metal ________________	*Roman ________________
medal ________________	*bell ________________

tap ’em ________________	*milk ________________
*totem ________________	golden ________________
gamble ________________	trickle ________________
gladdened ________________	patent ________________
Latin ________________	kitten ________________

Syllabic Consonants in Informal Speech

Transcription Exercise 3.4. Using Syllabics in Informal Speech

Some words in English have different pronunciations in formal and informal (casual) speech. Do not confuse informal with careless or sloppy speech. Transcribe each of these words with formal and informal pronunciations. Use syllabics in the informal transcriptions, but not in the formal. You should learn to hear and pronounce informal pronunciations even if you do not use them in your own speech.

Before proceeding, review the rule for homorganicity (item 6 in “Preliminaries for Transcribing Syllabics”). Then transcribe the first three words. For example, after /p/ and /b/, use syllabic /m/ and after /k/ and /g/, use syllabic /ŋ/. Check your transcriptions of the first five words with those provided in Appendix B of this workbook. When you understand the concept of the use of syllabics in informal speech, continue.

Formal Speech	Informal Speech
open ________________	________________
captain ________________	(“cap’n”) ________________
blacken ________________	________________
broken ________________	________________
napping ________________	________________
cabin ________________	________________
grabbing ________________	________________
milking ________________	________________
batting ________________	________________
ribbon ________________	________________

Audio-Activity 3.3. Listening for Syllabic Consonants (CD 1, Track 25)

Some of the eight words in this activity are spoken with a final syllabic, as in casual speech. Others are pronounced in a more formal style. Transcribe what you hear. Then check your answers.

1. ________	2. ________
3. ________	4. ________
5. ________	6. ________
7. ________	8. ________

Answers

ˈgoldn̩	ˈbɪdɪn
ˈkæpm̩	ˈgræbɪŋ
ˈnæpm̩	ˈopm̩
ˈopɪn	ˈmɪlkŋ̩

The Glottal Stop as a Variant of /t/ and /k/ Before a Syllabic

The glottal stop, /ʔ/, may serve as a variant of /t/ before /n̩/ and of /k/ before /ŋ̩/. (Its use before /l̩/ is found in such dialectal variations as /bɑʔl̩/ for *bottle*.) The /ʔ/ substitutes for the stop consonant and serves to turn off the vowel before the syllabic sound is made. There are other environments where the glottal stop is also found, such as when two stop consonants occur together within the same word: *nutcracker* (ˈnʌʔkrækɚ).

Transcription Exercise 3.5. The Glottal Stop

Transcribe these words, some of which you have seen before, using the glottal stop where possible. In those cases in which the glottal stop substitutes for a /t/, you will use a syllabic /n̩/ after the glottal stop. Where it replaces a /k/, you will use a syllabic /ŋ̩/.

kitten ________	patent ________
peltin' ________	broken ________
it blackened ________	bitten ________
molten ________	Latin ________
at Rome ________	combatant ________

Audio-Activity 3.4. Listening for the Glottal Stop (CD 1, Track 26)

Some of these words in this activity are pronounced with the glottal stop. If there is a glottal stop, transcribe it, along with the syllabic consonant following it. There are five words to transcribe. Check your answers.

1. ________ 2. ________
3. ________ 4. ________
5. ________

Answers

ˈkɪʔn̩	ˈlætɪn
ˈbroʔŋ̩	ˈpɛlʔn̩
ˈmolʔn̩	

A Dialect Variation: /ɛ/ to /ɪ/ Before a Nasal

In some dialects of American English, the letter *e* before a nasal consonant is pronounced /ɪ/ rather than /ɛ/. So the words *pin* and *pen* are both pronounced /pɪn/. The student should decide what his or her pronunciation of this vowel is before trying to transcribe the pronunciation of another dialect. It is necessary to be able to hear the difference even if one does not make that difference in speech.

Transcription Exercise 3.6. Transcribing /ɛ/ or /ɪ/

Using your dialect as a reference, transcribe the following words. If possible, listen to these words pronounced by a speaker of a dialect other than your own.

tinder ________	lender ________
tender ________	nimble ________
den ________	bent ________
din ________	grin ________
rental ________	penned ________
blend ________	meant ________
member ________	lemon ________
timber ________	limb ________

Audio-Activity 3.5. Listening for /ɪ/ and /ɛ/ (CD 1, Track 27)

Listen to these words and decide whether there is an /ɪ/ as in *pin*, or an /ɛ/ as in *pen* before the nasal sound. Then transcribe only the vowel. Some of the five items are nonsense. You do not have to transcribe the entire word. As usual, check your answers carefully.

1. ________ 2. ________
3. ________ 4. ________
5. ________

Answers

/ɛ/	/ɛ/
/ɛ/	/ɪ/
/ɪ/	

Audio-Activity 3.6. Listening and Transcribing /ɪ/ or /ɛ/ (CD 1, Track 28)

Transcribe these words as they are pronounced, paying attention to the vowel before the nasal. There are five items to transcribe.

1. ________ 2. ________
3. ________ 4. ________
5. ________

Answers

ə'tɛnd	'lɪmɪn
'bɛnt	'plɪnd
kən'tɛmd	

Loss of /t/ After /n/

In many dialects of American English, especially in informal speech, words like *winter* may be pronounced without the /t/ sound, so that *winter* sounds like *winner*. Notice that the /t/ is lost only when it follows a syllable with primary stress and either a vowel or syllabic consonant follows it. In *winter*, primary stress occurs on the first syllable (*win-*) and the reduced schwar (/ɚ/) follows /t/. In *entered*, for example, the /t/ may be lost, but not in *interred* (meaning "buried") because primary stress (the pitch jump) occurs on the last syllable.

Transcription Exercise 3.7. The Loss of /t/ in Informal Speech

Transcribe these words showing the loss of /t/ after /n/ in informal (conversational) speech. Pay close attention to what happens to your own pronunciation of the words listed. To avoid overpronouncing the words, you might imagine a sentence in a conversation to test your pronunciation more accurately. For example, for the first word in the list, you might imagine the sentence, "I believe he has a *mental* problem." Answers for the first six items in the left-hand column are provided in Appendix B of this workbook.

mental________________	mantle________________
memento________________	banter________________
planner________________	dented________________
planter________________	antler________________
(to) contend________________	lantern________________
pinto________________	bantam ________________
antic________________	canner________________
renter________________	canter________________
(to) contract________________	pander________________
rental________________	panic________________

Audio-Activity 3.7. Listening for the Loss of /t/ (CD 1, Track 29)

Transcribe the following, six words as they are pronounced, paying attention to the presence or absence of /t/.

1. ________ 2. ________
3. ________ 4. ________
5. ________ 6. ________

Answers

ˈpɪno	ˈlænɚn
ˈpændɚ	ˈrɛnl̩
ˈkɑnˈtrækt	ˈæntɪk

Transcribing /ɛ/ and /r/ in the Same Syllable

There are several vowels that can occur with /r/ in the same syllable. When this happens, they form a unit that must be learned for accuracy in transcription. The first of these vowel + /r/ combinations to be studied is /ɛr/ as in *air*. The primary mistake that students make in transcribing /ɛr/ is to use /er/ instead. However, /ɛr/ represents the sound better.

Transcription Exercise 3.8. Transcribing /ɛr/

Use the /ɛr/ combination where possible in the words that follow.

air ____________ bare ____________
care ____________ error ____________
wear ____________ glare ____________
mare ____________ pear ____________
blare ____________ bicker ____________

Transcribing Another Dialect Variation: /ɛ/ or /æ/ Before /r/

The pronunciation of vowels tends to change before /r/. One dialect variation of the vowel + /r/ combination is related to the sounds /ɛ/ and /æ/. If people pronounce both *marry* and *merry* with the same vowel, it is likely that they will use the vowel /ɛ/ in *both* words. If *marry* and *merry* are pronounced differently, it is probable that *marry* has /æ/ while *merry* has /ɛ/. The following exercise provides practice in transcribing these vowel + /r/ combinations.

Transcription Exercise 3.9. Transcribing /ɛ/ or /æ/ Before /r/

Transcribe the following words, noting any changes in the vowel before /r/. First, transcribe your own pronunciation, then transcribe the alternate pronunciation.

	My Pronunciation	Alternate Pronunciation
carom	____________	____________
clarinet	____________	____________
parent	____________	____________
carrot	____________	____________
marrow	____________	____________
arrow	____________	____________

Audio-Activity 3.8. Listening for /ɛ/ and /æ/ Before /r/ (CD 1, Track 30)

Review flash cards 28, 29, and 48. Write only the first vowel in each word that you hear to indicate the pronunciation of the vowel before /r/. There are six words. You do not have to transcribe the entire word.

		Answers	
1. ________	2. ________	/ɛ/	/æ/
3. ________	4. ________	/ɛ/	/ɛ/
5. ________	6. ________	/æ/	/æ/

Audio-Activity 3.9. Listening for and Transcribing /æ/ and /ɛ/ Before /r/ (CD 1, Track 31)

Transcribe these words, paying attention to the vowel before /r/ as pronounced. There are six words.

		Answers	
1. ________	2. ________	ˈpærət	ˈblɛr
3. ________	4. ________	ˈkærəm	ˈpɛrət
5. ________	6. ________	ˈæro	ˈɛrɚ

A Reexamination of /ŋ/

You have already learned that /ŋ/ occurs for the *ng* spelling in words like *tang, cling*, and *pang* as well as before *k* in words like *mink, tank*, and *twinkle* (see Transcription Exercise 2.6). For some words, such as *singer* and *hanger*, the spelling *ng* is transcribed /ŋ/. Usually such words have the *ng* spelling in the middle and are made up of a shorter word terminated with *ng* (*sing* and *hang*) to which another syllable (/ɚ/) is added. However, in words like *finger* and *anger*, the *ng* is transcribed /ŋg/. Notice that there is no shorter word, *fing* in *finger* or *ang* in *anger*. Therefore, the /ŋg/ pronunciation is used. There are exceptions to this rule, however. A few adjectives such as *longer* and *stronger* are pronounced with /ŋg/ although a shorter word appears in both (*long* and *strong*). It is therefore important to learn to hear the differences in sound rather than simply to rely on a rule.

Transcription Exercise 3.10. Transcribing /ŋ/

In transcribing the following words, do not use /e/ or /i/ in words like *angle* and *ankle*, or *ringer* and *tingle*. These pronunciations may exist in some dialects, but for the moment, use the most appropriate vowels that have been introduced so far in this text. The nasalization of the vowel, caused by influence from the velar nasal, often tricks us into thinking that /e/ and /i/ are the vowels of choice in such words, even though some speakers do use them.

The first two words in each column have been transcribed in Appendix B of this workbook so that you may check your own transcriptions.

angle________________	linking________________
ringer________________	dangled________________
linger________________	mingled________________
banging________________	wrinkle________________
ankle________________	tingle________________

Audio-Activity 3.10. Listening for /ŋ/ (CD 1, Track 32)

Transcribe the five words that you hear. Each contains /ŋ/.

1. ________ 2. ________
3. ________ 4. ________
5. ________

Answers

ˈræŋkl̩ ˈæŋgɚd
ˈrɪŋɪŋ ˈrɪŋkl̩
ˈlɪŋgɚ

Transcription Exercise 3.11. Marking Primary Stress in Three-Syllable Words

We have previously used the pitch test with words of two syllables. Recall that primary stress could occur on either the first syllable, as in *Tampa*, or the second, as in *canal*. In words of three syllables, primary stress may occur on either of the first two syllables, as in the words *TECHnical* or *roMANtic*. In this exercise, you will transcribe words of three syllables that fit these two patterns. First study the diagram illustrating the pitch test on the first word in each column. Then transcribe each of the remaining words, marking primary stress as appropriate.

Primary Stress on the First Syllable **Primary Stress on the Second Syllable**

Pitch Test:

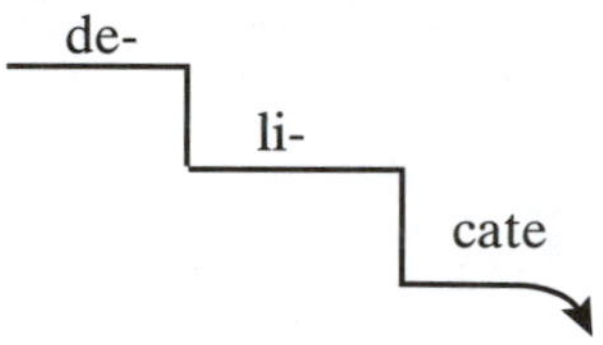

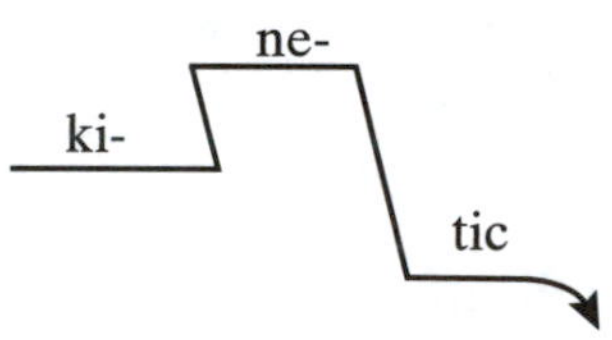

delicate____________________ kinetic____________________
radical____________________ poetic____________________
credible____________________ metallic____________________
democrat____________________ diploma____________________

More on Vowel Reduction: Vowel (or Syllable) Deletion

Another way in which vowels can be reduced occurs when, in unstressed syllables, they are lost completely. Similarly, syllabic consonants become nonsyllabic in such contexts. Pay close attention to item 3 in the following two examples:

A. 1. blacken		/blækən/	
2. blackened		/blækənd/	
3. blackening		/blækənɪŋ/	(no loss of /ə/)
	or	/blæknɪŋ/	(loss of /ə/)
B. 1. ripple		/rɪpl̩/	
2. rippled		/rɪpl̩d/	
3. rippling		/rɪpl̩ɪŋ/	(no loss of syllabic /l̩/)
	or	/rɪplɪŋ/	(loss of syllabic /l̩/)

In addition, speakers vary in their use of /ɚ/, especially when the following syllable begins with a vowel. Three pronunciations are observed. In the first, the /ɚ/ may retain its r-coloring. In the second, the /ɚ/ may become /ə/ and the /r/ may begin the next syllable. Finally, the vowel may be lost and the following syllable begins with /r/. Note example C.

C. 1. bicker		/ˈbɪkɚ/	(no vowel following)
2. bickered		/ˈbɪkɚd/	(no vowel following)
3. bickering		/ˈbɪkɚɪŋ/	(Case 1. /ɚ/ retained)
	or	/ˈbɪkərɪŋ/	(Case 2. /r/ releases the following syllable)
	or	/ˈbɪkrɪŋ/	(Case 3. Loss of vowel)

In situations like these, try to be consistent with your own speech or the speech of the person you are transcribing. Because all cases are appropriate for the language, your trained ear will tell you which form you should transcribe.

Transcription Exercise 3.12. Loss of Syllables

Using the principles that have been explained, transcribe the following words in their various forms.

a. Use syllabics in these words.

wrangle__________ wrangled__________

wrinkle__________ wrinkled__________

clamor__________ clamored__________

meddle__________ meddled__________

gladden__________ gladdened__________

crackle__________ crackled__________

b. Show retention of the syllabic before *-ing* in these words.

wrangling__________ wrinkling__________

clamoring__________ crackling__________

gladdening__________ meddling__________

c. Show loss of the syllablic before *-ing* in these words.

wrangling__________ wrinkling__________

clamoring__________ crackling__________

gladdening__________ meddling__________

Audio-Activity 3.11. Listening for the Presence or Absence of Syllabic Consonants (CD 1, Track 33)

Transcribe the four words that you hear, noting whether they are spoken with or without syllabic consonants.

1. ________ 2. ________

3. ________ 4. ________

Answers

ˈræŋgl̩ɪŋ	ˈtɪklɪŋ
ˈklæmbrɪŋ	ˈrɛkn̩nɪŋ

Transcription Exercise 3.13. Review

The following exercise will give you practice in transcribing various degrees of vowel reduction and stress placement in words of several syllables, as well as give you an opportunity to review the other principles of transcription learned so far. In transcribing these words, remember to mark primary stress appropriately. Your transcriptions of the first 10 items in the right-hand column may be compared to our answers by looking in Appendix B of this workbook.

dangling __________ canal__________

academic__________ maddening__________

pattering ______________________

timid ______________________

crackle ______________________

camera ______________________

calendar ______________________

minimum ______________________

opening ______________________

paneling ______________________

liberal ______________________

locale ______________________

reddening ______________________

romantic ______________________

abode ______________________

diplomatic ______________________

deadening ______________________

manacle ______________________

caroling ______________________

trampling ______________________

alpaca ______________________

Arabic ______________________

intellect ______________________

Manila ______________________

technical ______________________

peppering ______________________

pimento ______________________

pedantic ______________________

giggling ______________________

character ______________________

pragmatic ______________________

marimba ______________________

tepid ______________________

tantrum ______________________

Nolan ______________________

tandem ______________________

Audio-Activity 3.12. General Review (CD 1, Track 34)

This activity reviews the many principles of transcription covered so far. Be sure to show primary stress placement, syllabics, reduced vowels, alveolar flaps, and so on. There are 20 words.

1. ________ 2. ________
3. ________ 4. ________
5. ________ 6. ________
7. ________ 8. ________
9. ________ 10. ________
11. ________ 12. ________
13. ________ 14. ________
15. ________ 16. ________
17. ________ 18. ________
19. ________ 20. ________

Answers

kɪ'nɛɾɪk	'krɛdəbl̩
'tɪmɪd	ə'bod
pə'dænɪk	'gɪgl̩ɪŋ
'tæntrəm	'rɛdnɪŋ
'kærəktɚ	'kɛrl̩ɪŋ
po'ɛt̬ɪk	'træmplɪŋ
'ɪnəlɛkt	'tɛpɪd
'opm̩nɪŋ	'pæt̬ɚɪŋ
'ɛrəbɪk	pə'mɛnto
'pɛprɪŋ	'tændəm

Transcription Exercise 3.14. Optional Advanced Transcription

aloof ______________________

dozen ______________________

mix ______________________

hoax ______________________

union ______________________

deacon ______________________

behavior ______________________

youth ______________________

welcome____________________

aware____________________

wallet____________________

Yiddish____________________

stallion____________________

yodler____________________

worship____________________

phlegm____________________

Wisconsin____________________

heath____________________

sparrow____________________

hermit____________________

inhale____________________

gangway____________________

rockers ____________________

Paris ____________________

lugged ____________________

whopper____________________

SECTION 4

Consonants: /j, w, h/
Vowels and Diphthong: /ʌ, ɝ, ɑ, u, ju/

Learning Activities: An Introduction to the Sounds in Section 4

Learning Activity 4.1. The Glides and Fricative /h/

Read about the glides /j/ and /w/ in Chapter 9 of *Applied Phonetics* (*AP*) (p. 187). The fricative /h/ is found in Chapter 6 (p. 150) Then fill in the blanks in the following Learning Activity.

1. What is meant by the term "glide?"____________________
2. /j/ and /w/ are glides. Are they offglides or onglides? ____________________
3. What is the symbol for the voiced bilabial glide? ____________________
4. For non-native speakers of English, it is important to emphasize ____________ in producing the /w/ sound.
5. What is the symbol for the voiced palatal glide?____________________
6. What is the symbol for the voiceless glottal fricative? ____________________
7. In *AP*, there is no articulatory diagram or palatogram for /h/. Why? ____________________
   ____
8. Some phoneticians consider the /h/ to be an on- ____________________.

Learning Activity 4.2. More Vowels and a Diphthong: /ʌ, ɝ, u, ɑ, ju/

Read about vowels and diphthongs in Chapters 11, 12, and 13 in *Applied Phonetics*. After reviewing these sounds, complete the following Learning Activity by filling in the blanks.

1. Provide the symbol for the descriptions or names of the sounds in this section.
   a. the diphthong: ____________________
   b. the caret: ____________________
   c. the reversed-hooked epsilon (or stressed schwar): ____________________
   d. the high back tense vowel: ____________________

e. the unrounded back vowel: ____________________
f. the central vowel: ____________________
g. the r-colored vowel: ____________________

2. In this list, what is the most frequently used vowel in English speech? (See Appendix B in *AP*, page, 341) ________

3. According to Dewey (1971), how many different spellings in English are there for:

/ɑ/: ________
/u/: ________
/ʌ/: ________
/ju/: ________
/ɝ/: ________

Learning to Transcribe These Sounds: Consonants: /j, w, h/ Vowels and a Diphthong: /ʌ, ɝ, ɑ, u, ju/

Introduction

The consonants /j/, /h/, and /w/ do not occur in word-final position, but only in initial or medial position. Remembering that these sounds have an onglide rather than an offglide character will help in avoiding the use of these sounds at the ends of words or before other consonants within words. Each sound is used as a transition to a vowel and not as a means of leaving a vowel sound. With few exceptions, the transcription of these sounds is clear.

The /j/ as in *Yes*

Perhaps the selection of this symbol by the International Phonetic Association (IPA) was the result of Germanic influence from such important early phoneticians as Otto Jespersen. Under such influence, /j/ was selected instead of /y/ for this sound. The name given to this symbol is *jod* (or *yod*).

Transcription Exercise 4.1. Transcribing /j/

Pay special attention to the use of this sound as a glide.

yak ____________	yet ____________
yellow ____________	yank ____________
yelp ____________	yokel ____________
Yo-Yo ____________	canyon ____________
million ____________	yogurt ____________
billiard ____________	yodel ____________

The /h/ as in *Hoe*

Transcription Exercise 4.2. Transcribing /h/

hammock ____________	Homer ____________
habitat ____________	hidden ____________
ahem ____________	ahead ____________

hymnal________________	inhibit________________
heckle________________	Hank________________
yo-ho-ho________________	halibut________________

The /w/ as in *Woe*

Transcription Exercise 4.3. Transcribing /w/

welcome________________	wing________________
landward________________	windmill________________
quack________________	Gwendolyn________________
quintet________________	tranquil________________
quick-witted________________	William________________
twang________________	twitter________________
wicker________________	quicken________________

Audio-Activity 4.1. Listening for /j/, /h/, *and* /w/ *(CD 1, Track 35)*

Review the material in Transcription Exercises 4.1, 4.2, and 4.3, and locate flash cards 15, 21, and 22. Transcribe only the *first* sound in each of these six words. Check your answers when finished.

		Answers	
1. ________	2. ________	/j/	/h/
3. ________	4. ________	/w/	/j/
5. ________	6. ________	/h/	/w/

The /hw/: Do You Use It in *Which?*

Originally, the spelling *wh* stood for the combination of sounds that can best be transcribed in IPA symbols as /hw/. In various regions, the /hw/ sound has been lost and *wh* most frequently spells the pronunciation of the sound /w/. Among some speakers, however, the /hw/ sound has been retained; for them, *what* differs in pronunciation from *watt*. An alternate symbol for this sound is /ʍ/.

Transcription Exercise 4.4. Transcribing /hw/

Practice transcribing and producing the /hw/ where appropriate in the following words, even if you do not produce /hw/ in your own speech. One word of caution is in order: Use great care when you transcribe the speech of others because many speakers do not use the /hw/ in their speech. Do not be misled by English orthography. The answers to the first four words in the lefthand column are provided in Appendix B of this workbook.

whelp________________	whittle________________
wet________________	whet________________
whim________________	whit________________
where________________	wear________________
hack________________	whack________________

Audio-Activity 4.2. Listening for /w/, /h/, *and* /hw/ *(CD 1, Track 36)*

For this activity transcribe /w/, /h/, or /hw/ as appropriate for these words. Some of these six items contain more than one of these three sounds. You do not have to transcribe the entire word, but only the required symbol(s).

		Answers	
1. ________	2. ________	/hw/	/w/, /h/
3. ________	4. ________	/hw/	/h/, /w/, /hw/
5. ________	6. ________	/hw/, /w/	/w/

Audio-Activity 4.3. Contrasting /w/ *and* /hw/ *(CD 1, Track 37)*

Now transcribe these pairs of words just as they are spoken. Remember that they may not be pronounced the same in your speech. There are six words.

		Answers	
1. ________	2. ________	ˈhwɪtʃ	ˈwɪtʃ
3. ________	4. ________	ˈwɛr	ˈhwɛr
5. ________	6. ________	ˈhwɛt	ˈwɛt

The Vowel /ɑ/ as in *Father*

The /ɑ/ sound is often represented orthographically with the letter *o* as in *mop*. Once the sound-symbol association is made, students have little problem transcribing this common vowel.

Transcription Exercise 4.5. Transcribing /ɑ/

model ____________________	wander ____________________
hopper ____________________	knot ____________________
hypnotic ____________________	collar ____________________
locker ____________________	pompom ____________________
dollop ____________________	dole ____________________
waddle ____________________	hotter ____________________

The /ɑ/ + /r/ Combination as in *Far*

The next vowel + /r/ combination that you will learn to transcribe is /ɑr/. This combination does not cause undue problems for beginning transcribers who have this sound in their dialect (see Transcription Exercise 4.9).

Transcription Exercise 4.6. Transcribing /ɑr/

armored ____________________	tar ____________________
car hop ____________________	market ____________________
heart ____________________	article ____________________
yard ____________________	bargain ____________________
depart ____________________	artist ____________________

Audio-Activity 4.4. Listening for /ɑ/ and /ɑr/ (CD 1, Track 38)

Transcribe these five words containing /ɑ/ and /ɑr/. One nonsense item is included.

1. ________ 2. ________
3. ________ 4. ________
5. ________

Answers

hɪpˈnɑt̬ɪk ˈɑfl̩
ˈpɑm pɑm ˈɑrmɚd
pɑˈtɑkɑlə

Contrasting /ə/ and /ʌ/—The Neutral Vowels as in *Above*

You studied the reduced, neutral schwa vowel in Section 2. American English also has a stressed version of the same vowel—the caret or /ʌ/. It is always found in stressed syllables and is therefore used less frequently than the schwa. (If you are unclear on the concept of stress [emphasis], read Part I, Section 7 of this workbook at this time.) The /ʌ/ sound is heard in the word *hut*. In some variations of the IPA, the schwa symbol is used for both the stressed and the unstressed sounds, so that both vowels in a word like *abut* would be transcribed with identical symbols. As used in this text, *abut* will be transcribed /ə ˈbʌt/. It is wise for the student to consider /ʌ/ as a standard phoneme of English with /ə/ being most frequently used as a reduced form of it or another vowel.

Transcription Exercise 4.7. The Neutral Vowels

Transcribe these words emphasizing the difference between /ʌ/ and /ə/.

a cut________	onion________
yucca________	muddle________
wonder________	humbug________
color________	puppet________
young________	bunion________
couple________	grumble________
a knot________	a ton________

Audio-Activity 4.5. Listening for Neutral Vowels (CD 1, Track 39)

Locate flash cards 30 and 31 and place them in front of you. Point to the one found in each of the items that you will hear. Then transcribe the appropriate vowel (but not the entire word). Learn to listen for the stressed syllable. There are six items, including two non-words.

1. ________ 2. ________
3. ________ 4. ________
5. ________ 6. ________

This is the end of CD 1.

Answers

/ʌ/ /ə/
/ə/ /ʌ/
/ə/ /ʌ/

Contrasting the R-Colored Vowels: /ɝ/ and /ɚ/ as in *Herder*

The reversed hooked epsilon, also called the stressed schwar, (/ɝ/), is the stressed version of /ɚ/ and is therefore found only in stressed syllables. In transcription, it tends to be slightly less frequent than /ɚ/, which may serve as a reduced form of /ɝ/. A variant transcription practice is to use the schwa /ə/ followed by /r/ for both the stressed and unstressed versions of this sound. Our practice is to differentiate between these two very similar sounds so that *myrrh* is transcribed as /ˈmɝ/ and *murder* appears as /ˈmɝdɚ/.

Transcription Exercise 4.8. The R-Colored Vowels

Transcribe, making a distinction between /ɝ/ and /ɚ/. Should your dialect lack these sounds, practice using them here.

yearn ____________	girder ____________
grammar ____________	Burton ____________
twirled ____________	worker ____________
entered ____________	interred ____________
Merlin ____________	blurb ____________
polar ____________	world ____________
limerick ____________	were ____________
admiral ____________	quirk ____________
clobber ____________	blubber ____________

Audio-Activity 4.6. Listening for /ɝ/ and /ɚ/ (CD 2, Track 1)

With this Audio-Activity, we begin the second of the CDs that accompany this workbook. Review flash cards 32 and 33. When you are ready, transcribe these six items, including the nonsense words. Check your answers with those provided.

1. ________ 2. ________
3. ________ 4. ________
5. ________ 6. ________

Answers

ˈtwɝld	ˈwɝd
ˈblɑt̬ɚ	ˈlɝklo
ˈgɝdɚ	ˈklolɚ

A Dialect Variation: R-Dropping

In some dialects, especially Southern American, there is a tendency to drop the /r/ when it follows certain vowels. In such dialects, the /ɝ/ sound does not regularly occur. Instead, a vowel without r-coloring is used. The symbol is the reversed epsilon without the hook that signifies r-coloring (/ɜ/). For example, *bird* is not pronounced /bɝd/, but rather /bɜd/. At times, one also hears a diphthongization of /ɜ/ so that /bɜd/ is pronounced /bɜ͜ɪd/. Frequently, this variation is perceived as *boyd*, but this pronunciation is rare. In unstressed positions, the schwa without the hook is used to show lack of r-coloring.

Transcription Exercise 4.9. R-Dropping in Southern American Dialect

Transcribe these words, using /ɜ/ and /ə/ to show the loss of r-coloring. Compare the pronunciation of these words to their counterparts in Transcription Exercise 4.8. Appendix B of this workbook provides the answers for the first four words in the left-hand column.

yearn ____________	girder ____________
entered ____________	worker ____________
Merlin ____________	blurb ____________
polar ____________	quirk ____________
clobber ____________	blubber ____________

Audio-Activity 4.7. Listening for Alternate Pronunciations (CD 2, Track 2)

Review Transcription Exercise 4.9, then listen to these four pairs of words and transcribe each as pronounced. There are eight words, including two non-words.

1. ________ 2. ________
3. ________ 4. ________
5. ________ 6. ________
7. ________ 8. ________

Answers

ˈpæt̬ɚ	ˈpæt̬ə
ˈblɝbɚ	ˈblɜbə
ˈjɜn	ˈjɝn
ˈɝbən	ˈɜbən

The Vowel /u/ as in *Boo*

The vowel /u/ is not usually a problem sound to transcribe as long as we remember that it is pronounced as a single sound and not as its alphabet letter: /j͜u/ (see Transcription Exercise 4.11). It is often represented in regular spelling by *oo* as in *too, boot*, and *hoot*.

Transcription Exercise 4.10. Transcribing /u/

boot ________	grew ________
moot ________	lunar ________
brutal ________	who ________
canoe ________	burner ________
poodle ________	group ________
Lou ________	bluegill ________

The Diphthong /j͜u/ as in *You*

The /j/ sound, which was already discussed, can also serve as an onglide to the high back vowel /u/. Compare *moo* and *mew*, /mu/ and /mj͜u/. In spelling, the single letter *u* may stand for both components of this diphthong. In transcribing, do not forget to use a *slue*, the curved line placed under this distinctive (phonemic) diphthong, to show that both elements of this sound occur in the same syllable.

Transcription Exercise 4.11. Transcribing the /j͜u/ Diphthong

yoo-hoo ________	butte ________
mute ________	you ________
Hugh ________	too few ________
cue ________	puke ________
unit ________	cube ________
human ________	whom ________

Audio-Activity 4.8. Listening for /u/ and /j͜u/ (CD 2, Track 3)

Locate flash cards 34 and 42 to provide visual feedback for you as you listen to these six items and transcribe each completely. There is one nonsense item.

1. ________ 2. ________
3. ________ 4. ________
5. ________ 6. ________

Answers

ˈlunɚ	ˈhu
ˈbj͜ut	tu ˈfj͜u
ˈhj͜u	ˈtj͜u bu

The Diphthong /ju͜/ After Labials and Alveolars

Originally in English, the spelling *u* or *ew* was pronounced /ju͜/. The pronunciation of this diphthong is stable after the labials /m, b, p, v, f/ as in *music, beauty, pew, view*, and *few*, and usually after the velars /k/ and /g/ as in *cue* and *argue*. However, in General American English, this pronunciation has simplified to /u/ after the alveolar consonants /l/ and /s/ as in *lute* and *suit*. After the alveolar consonants /t, d, n/, *u* or *ew* may be pronounced /ju͜/ or /u/. For example, compare these pronunciations of *new*: /nju͜/ or /nu/.

Transcription Exercise 4.12. Transcribing /ju͜/ or /u/

Use your own dialect as your reference. Check your answers to the first three items in each column in Appendix B.

tune ________	cartoon ________
cute ________	yew ________
nude ________	noodle ________
mooing ________	mewing ________
knew ________	noon ________
dune ________	doom ________
dew ________	do ________

Audio-Activity 4.9. Listening for Alternate Pronunciations (CD 2, Track 4)

Complete Transcription Exercise 4.12 first. Then listen for different pronunciations in the five words that you will hear. Transcribe each, then check your answers.

1. ________ 2. ________
3. ________ 4. ________
5. ________

Answers

ˈtju͜n	ˈnu
kɑrˈtun	ˈnju͜
ˈtun	

Transcription Exercise 4.13. Review Transcription

The first six items in each column are transcribed in Appendix B of this workbook so that you may check your work.

ha-ha ________	herb ________
Curt ________	wad ________
young ________	pucker ________
wand ________	purr ________
her ________	a block ________
her pen ________	crumb ________
whom ________	hewn ________
hue ________	bugle ________
burned ________	woo ________
union ________	mogul ________
yacht ________	yoga ________
grotto ________	wigwam ________

yelling ________	blurt ________
crouton ________	wicked ________
Newton ________	pocket ________
twirp ________	supper ________
column ________	quota ________
blood ________	noggin ________
curtain ________	human ________
operatic ________	hamburger ________
whimpering ________	hobble ________
pollen ________	yodel ________
billion ________	network ________
cubic ________	common ________
whirlwind ________	hallelujah ________
wiggle ________	Yule ________

Audio-Activity 4.10. Auditory Review (CD 2, Track 5)

Transcribe these 10 words as pronounced.

1. ________	2. ________
3. ________	4. ________
5. ________	6. ________
7. ________	8. ________
9. ________	10. ________

Answers

'pʌdl̩	'blɜt
hælə'lujə	'hwɪmpɚɪŋ
'jɑt	'bj͜ugl̩
'hæmbɚgɚ	'hj͜umɪn
'pʌkɚ	ɑpə'ræt̬ɪk

Transcription Exercise 4.14. Optional Advanced Transcription

The multisyllabic words in this exercise contain some of the sounds yet to be introduced in this text.

kumquat ________	translation ________
dictation ________	gyroscope ________
discussion ________	skyscraper ________
organizer ________	magnify ________
scholastic ________	Jupiter ________
smithereens ________	togetherness ________
thrilling ________	vegetarian ________
ivory ________	equator ________
squadron ________	zodiac ________
newsprint ________	vanity ________
interview ________	Russell ________
reinforce ________	procured ________
afterbirth ________	atmosphere ________

SECTION 5

Consonants: /s, z, ʃ, ʒ, f, v/
Vowels and Diphthongs: /e, ʊ, a͜ɪ, ɔ͜ɪ/

■ Learning Activities: An Introduction to the Sounds in Section 5

Learning Activity 5.1. The Sibilants: /s, z, ʃ, ʒ/

Read about these sounds in Chapter 6 of *Applied Phonetics* (*AP*) (pp. 129–155). Then provide the symbols for sounds described in this learning activity.

1. The voiceless palatal fricative: ____________
2. The voiceless alveolar fricative: ____________
3. The stretched s: ____________
4. The voiced palatal fricative: ____________
5. The voiced alveolar fricative: ____________
6. Which two symbols may be used to transcribe the plural morpheme in English? ____________
7. The letter *s* represents this sound 64% of the time that the sound occurs: ____________
8. The letter *s* represents this sound 73% of the time that the sound occurs: ____________
9. The letter *s* represents this sound 33% of the time that the sound occurs: ____________
10. Which of these sounds does not occur in word initial position in American English? ________

Learning Activity 5.2. Short Answer

1. Why are the sounds /s, z, ʃ, ʒ/ described as "grooved?" ____________
____
____
2. What does the term "sibilant" mean? ____________
____

Learning Activity 5.3. The Fricatives: /f, v/

Read about these two sounds in Chapter 6 of *AP* (pp. 109–119). Then answer these questions.

1. What is the phonetic symbol for the voiceless labiodental fricative? ____________________
2. What is the symbol for the voiced labiodental fricative? ____________________
3. What is the active articulator for /f/ and /v/? ____________________
4. What is the passive articulator for /f/ and /v/? ____________________
5. Is the velopharyngeal port opened or closed for the production of these sounds? ____________________

Learning Activity 5.4. More Vowels and Two Diphthongs: /e, ʊ, a͜ɪ, ɔ͜ɪ/

Read about these vowels and diphthongs in Chapters 10 (p. 228), 12 (p. 276), and 13 (pp. 301, 314) of *AP*. Then complete the following by providing the phonetic symbol for the sound that is described.

1. The lower high back lax vowel: ____________________
2. The mid-front tense vowel: ____________________
3. The "flying u": ____________________
4. The mid-back-to-high-front diphthong: ____________________
5. The low-front-to-high-front diphthong: ____________________
6. The diphthong that used the "capped a" in its description: ____________________
7. The cardinal vowel in this series: ____________________
8. In addition to the two diphthongs in this series, the sound that is frequently transcribed as a diphthong:
____

Learning to Transcribe These Sounds: Consonants: /s, z, ʃ, ʒ, f, v/ Vowels and Diphthongs: /e, ʊ, a͜ɪ, ɔ͜ɪ/

Introduction

The consonants, vowels, and diphthongs in this set are slightly more difficult to master than those presented before because there are five new symbol configurations to learn along with a new sound value that corresponds to the alphabet letter *e*. Except for some of their allophonic variations, /s/, /z/, /f/, and /v/ should not cause undue problem for the transcriber.

The Sibilants: /s, z, ʃ, ʒ/ as in *Sip, Zip, Mesher*, and *Measure*

The sounds in this group are called sibilants, which means "hissing." Some phoneticians also include the affricates /tʃ/ as in *chew* and /dʒ/ as in *Jew* with the sibilants, but they will be introduced later. The /s/ and /z/, found in the words *Sue* and *zoo*, are not new symbols. However, /ʃ/ and /ʒ/, as in *Asher* and *azure*, are new and the transcriber must remember to stretch both symbols so that they extend below most of the other phonetic symbols in much the same way as /j/. The /ʒ/ is not a very common sound in English and therefore the opportunities to transcribe it are limited. Note that words such as *notion* and *pleasure* are not transcribed with the /j/ following /ʃ/ or /ʒ/. Some phoneticians prefer to write the /ʃ/ as /š/ and the /ʒ/ as /ž/ (called either s-wedge/z-wedge or s-check/z-check). In this text, the authorized International Phonetic Association (IPA) symbols are used.

Transcription Exercise 5.1. Transcribing the Sibilants

Check your transcriptions for the first six words in the right-hand column in Appendix B.

sap________	zap________
zipper ________	sipper________
shop________	whiz________
wish________	garage________
sit________	treasure________
crash________	ruts________
worst________	Zen________
pleasure________	casts________
Russia________	windowsill________
ship________	newsprint________
czar________	shimmer________
azure________	shipwrecked ________
shinbone ________	zigzagging________
slowed________	pleasurable________
skillets________	bombshell________
notion ________	bonanza________
pessimist________	snow boots________
zip code ________	buzzer________
workshop________	allusion________
measuring________	cosmopolitan________

Audio-Activity 5.1. Listening for the Sibilants in Non-Words (CD 2, Track 6)

Locate flash cards 11, 12, 13, and 14 and complete Transcription Exercises 5.1. Then transcribe the following eight nonsense items containing these new sounds. Check your answers with those provided.

		Answers	
1. ______	2. ______	ˈsæzə	ˈʒæʃə
3. ______	4. ______	ˈzɪmz	ˈʃɑs
5. ______	6. ______	pəˈʒɪzə	ˈbj͜uʒ
7. ______	8. ______	səˈsʌʃə	ˈʒɪʃɑ

Audio-Activity 5.2. Listening for the Sibilants in Common Words (CD 2, Track 7)

Here are six words containing various sibilants. Transcribe them completely, noting how /s/ may serve to mark plurality (see Transcription Exercise 5.3).

		Answers	
1. ______	2. ______	gəˈrɑʒ	ˈplɛʒɚəbl̩
3. ______	4. ______	ˈʃæmrɑks	ˈstj͜udn̩ts
5. ______	6. ______	ˈwɪndəsɪl	ˈpɛsəmɪst

Devoicing of Final-Position /z̥/

Many speakers of American English may devoice /z/ when it ends a word, occurs before a pause, or is followed by a voiceless consonant. In words that end with a voiced consonant and orthographic *s*, the convention is to transcribe with /z/. However, what is said by many speakers is actually a partially devoiced /z/ or a /z̥/ that starts as /z/ but ends as /s/. The diacritic for devoicing or partial devoicing is a small circle placed under the symbol, /z̥/. In transcription, the devoicing of /z/ requires this diacritic.

Transcription Exercise 5.2. The Devoicing of /z̥/

Transcribe, using the diacritic to show the devoicing of /z/ where appropriate. You may check your transcription of the first six words in the left-hand column with the transcription provided in Appendix B.

cones__________	grows__________
pose__________	commas__________
buzz__________	Bob's__________
cobwebs__________	sheds__________
runs__________	amuse__________
snooze__________	disclose__________
Liz__________	tubes__________
discovers__________	carnivals__________

Audio-Activity 5.3. Listening for the Devoicing of /z/ (CD 2, Track 8)

Review Transcription Exercise 5.2 on the devoicing of final position /z/. Transcribe these six words completely. In checking your answers, pay attention to the use of the diacritic for devoicing.

1. ________	2. ________
3. ________	4. ________
5. ________	6. ________

Answers

ˈgroz̥	məˈrɑʒɪz̥
ˈɛpəsodz̥	ˈbɑbz̥
ˈkɑbwɛbz̥	ˈsɪzɚz̥

The Sibilants as Grammatical Markers

The /s/ and /z/ serve important grammatical functions in the English language. They do extra work as plural and possessive morpheme markers as in *cats* and *cat's*. They also signal the third person on verbs, as in *John runs*. Because only *s* is used in spelling, students of phonetics may not be sure when the plural, possessive, or third person marker should be transcribed /s/ or /z/. Nevertheless, in most cases, knowing a simple rule will keep you from making needless mistakes. When a word ends in a voiced consonant or vowel, use /z/; when a word ends in a voiceless consonant, use /s/; and when a word ends in a sibilant (or affricate), add another syllable—either /əz/ or /ɪz/, depending on your preference. Do not forget to mark the final-position /z/ for devoicing, as shown in Transcription Exercise 5.2.

Transcription Exercise 5.3. Grammatical Markers

Transcribe these words. Notice the grammatical role of the sibilants. Use the rule as stated above to help you in any ambiguous cases that arise. The first five words in both columns are transcribed in Appendix B so that you can make sure that you are on the right track.

knocks__________	boxes__________
ceramics__________	echoes__________
student's__________	bibs__________

dishes ______________
Tom's ______________
docks ______________
presses ______________
comas ______________
shocks ______________
comics ______________
slopes ______________
episodes ______________
sunglasses ______________
shamrocks ______________
albums ______________
wishes ______________

mirages ______________
Alice's ______________
attacks ______________
brushes ______________
gallows ______________
roughes ______________
heads ______________
gum drops ______________
precipices ______________
reciprocals ______________
snows ______________
scissors ______________
brans ______________

The /n/ and /s/ Problem: *Prince* or *Prints?*

Compare your pronunciation of the words *prince* and *prints*. Because they are pronounced essentially the same by many speakers, the question is whether they should be transcribed differently: /prɪns/ or /prɪnts/. If words are pronounced identically, they should be transcribed to show the similarity. We, therefore, recommend using /nts/ for words having the *nts* letter combination, such as *prints*; and /n^{t}s/, with a raised *t*, for words having the *ns* combination. This convention applies only to these sound combinations within the same syllable. When the *n* ends one syllable and the *s* begins the next, as in *insect* (*in-sect*), the intrusive *t* may not occur. However, speakers of American English may use a /t/ prior to the s-release in some words. For example, pay attention to your pronunciation of *answer* in the set of words in Transcription Exercise 5.4.

Transcription Exercise 5.4. Transcribing "ns" *Combinations*

Not all of the words in this exercise require the intrusive *t*. Remember to raise the intrusive *t* in words that do not have the letter *t* in their spelling. The first three words in each column are transcribed in Appendix B of this workbook.

sense ______________
cents ______________
mints ______________
consume ______________
presence ______________
France ______________
dense ______________
balance ______________

scents ______________
insect ______________
mince ______________
incompetence ______________
presents ______________
instrumental ______________
dents ______________
answer ______________

Audio-Activity 5.4. Listening for "ns" *Combinations (CD 2, Track 9)*

This activity provides experience in listening for *ns* or *nts* combinations as you did in Transcription Exercise 5.4. Transcribe the following six items. For the two nonsense words, do not lift the /t/ above the other symbols. Check your work when finished.

1. ________	2. ________		
3. ________	4. ________		
5. ________	6. ________		

Answers

'æn^{t}sɚ	prə'sænts
'bælɪn^{t}s	'ʃæprənts
'ænsɚ	kən'dɛn^{t}s

The Vowel /e/ as in *Way*

The /e/ sound is a tense front vowel that is not pronounced as its "letter value" in the English alphabet (i.e., as /i/). Speakers of American English often diphthongize it in stressed and open syllables, that is, syllables not closed by a consonant—as in *bay* /be͜ɪ/. As a result, it is often transcribed /e͜ɪ/. If your teacher so directs, use the diphthongized version for transcribing this sound in stressed or open syllables. Otherwise, use /e/. Due to the fact that no English words are contrasted on the basis of whether or not the /e/ is diphthongized, there is little reason to use the /e͜ɪ/ in a broad or phonemic transcription. It is useful in narrower or allophonic transcriptions, however.

Transcription Exercise 5.5. Practice With /e/ as in Way

Transcribe these words using /e/ (or /e͜ɪ) where appropriate. The first four words in each column are included in Appendix B of this workbook so that you may check your work, if necessary. You should have less need for Appendix B by now.

aide________________	player________________
eight________________	nation________________
paced________________	pest________________
attain________________	locate________________
belt ________________	built ________________
open________________	amaze ________________
cape________________	greater________________
state________________	no way________________
contemplate________________	brainstem ________________
meditate________________	April________________
Asia________________	wallpaper ________________
accommodate ________________	sensational ________________
impatience ________________	patients________________

Audio-Activity 5.5. Listening for /e/ (CD 2, Track 10)

Locate and study flash card 27 and complete Transcription Exercise 5.5. Then transcribe the following six items completely. The last two are nonsense words.

1. ________	2. ________
3. ________	4. ________
5. ________	6. ________

Answers

'eprl̩	ə'kɑmədet
sɛn'seʃənl̩	'peʃənts ~ -n^{t}s
'eʃl̩	brə'sepələ

The Consonants /f/ and /v/ as in *Fan* and *Van*

The labiodental sounds /f/ and /v/, as in *fan* and *van*, are fairly straightforward with regard to their transcription. Contrasted with the grooved fricative sibilants, the /f/ and /v/ form part of a set of fricative sounds known as slit fricatives because of the narrow opening formed by the lips and teeth.

Transcription Exercise 5.6. Transcribing /f/ and /v/

face ______	foam ______
fence ______	phonic ______
affirm ______	vague ______
valor ______	diffused ______
converse ______	artifact ______
offensive ______	devastate ______
toughen ______	forgiven ______
infallible ______	slave ______
waterproof ______	photograph ______
enough ______	waffle ______
approval ______	flashback ______
revolver ______	inflatable ______
expensive ______	unmerciful ______
captive ______	laugh ______
vacation ______	freshman ______
nervous ______	starved ______
afterglow ______	frivolous ______

Audio-Activity 5.6. Listening for /f/ and /v/ (CD 2, Track 11)

This activity is based on Transcription Exercise 5.6 and flash cards 7 and 8. There are six items in this list, including two non-words.

1. ______	2. ______
3. ______	4. ______
5. ______	6. ______

Answers

ˈfot̬əgræf	rəˈmuvl̩
ɪnˈfæləbl̩	ˈfrɪvələs
ˈvæfəvə	ˈflɑvnɪf

The Loss of /t/ After the Fricatives /f/ or /s/

Previously, you learned that the /t/ sound may not be pronounced in words such as *winter* or *antic* (see Transcription Exercise 3.7). It may also not be pronounced in certain words in which /t/ occurs after /f/ as in *often* or *soften* and /s/ as in *thistle* or *bustle*. Closer analysis reveals that this change may be caused by assimilation, as in *left field*, in which the /f/ sound in the first syllable blends with the same sound in the second syllable, resulting in the loss of /t/. On other occasions, the homorganic nature of the sounds (/s, t, l, n/ are alveolar) cause the loss of /t/ after the fricative /s/. Finally, the /t/ may be omitted because of the difficult nature of producing all the sounds in a phonotactic environment (*investment* or *craft class*).

Transcription Exercise 5.7. The Loss of /t/

Transcribe these words showing the loss of /t/ following /s/ or /f/.

wrestle__________	investment__________
christen__________	hustle__________
left shoe__________	nestle__________
mistletoe__________	craft class __________
shiftless__________	apostle __________

The Shift From /v/ to /b/ Before Syllabic /m̩/ in Informal Speech

The transcriber should be aware that at times in informal speech, the /v/ may shift to a /b/ (a voiced bilabial stop) before /m̩/, as in *have 'em* (/hæbm̩/). Compare this pronounciation to the more formal /ˈhævəm/.

Transcription Exercise 5.8. Practicing the /v/ *to* /b/ *Shift*

Transcribe these items in two ways—formally and informally. The answers to the first two words are provided in Appendix B of this workbook.

	Formal Speech	Informal [/-bm̩/] Speech
driven	__________	__________
eleven	__________	__________
serve 'em	__________	__________
government	__________	__________
heaven	__________	__________
ovenware	__________	__________
seven	__________	__________
haven't	__________	__________

Audio-Activity 5.7. Listening for the /v/ *to* /b/ *Shift (CD 2, Track 12)*

Review Transcription Exercise 5.8 then decide which are the formal and informal pronunciations in the following pairs of words that you will hear, and transcribe accordingly. In this list of six words, the last two are nonsensical.

1. ________ 2. ________
3. ________ 4. ________
5. ________ 6. ________

Answers

əˈlɛvən	əˈlɛbm̩
ˈhɛbm̩	ˈhɛvɪn
ˈpæbm̩ʃɑ	ˈpævɪnʃɑ

The Vowel /ʊ/ as in *Hood*

The vowel /ʊ/ is found in some very common English words, such as *good, book, cook,* and *push,* but otherwise it does not occur very frequently. It is made similarly to the stressed /ʌ/ except that the lips are rounded. Students find the similarity between the two symbols for the high back vowels, /u/ and /ʊ/, helpful in learning to distinguish between them in transcribing speech.

Transcription Exercise 5.9. Transcribing /ʊ/

The first three items in each column are transcribed in Appendix B of this workbook should you need to check your transcription of this sound.

should ____________	sugar ____________
booking ____________	shook ____________
look ____________	luck ____________
woman ____________	goodness ____________
fulfillment ____________	stood ____________
could ____________	input ____________
foot ____________	heard ____________
hood ____________	wood ____________
Luke ____________	pushes ____________
cooled ____________	nook ____________
casual ____________	sensual ____________

Common Vowel Change Affecting /u/ and /ʊ/

Wise (1957) reports that in all dialects, especially those of the Eastern United States, a shift from /u/ to /ʊ/ may occur in words written with *oo*. Although the words *pool* and *book* are almost always pronounced /pul/ and /bʊk/, the pronunciation of some other words is more flexible. Wise suggests that, when there is doubt about how to pronounce one of these words, it is safe to use /u/.

Transcription Exercise 5.10. Transcribing Words with /u/ *and* /ʊ/

Practice pronouncing the words in this exercise both ways. Which is your preference?

/u/	/ʊ/
hoop ____________	____________
roof ____________	____________
Cooper ____________	____________
groom ____________	____________
root ____________	____________
soot ____________	____________
room ____________	____________
broom ____________	____________

Audio-Activity 5.8. Listening for /u/ *and* /ʊ/ *(CD 2, Track 13)*

Once mastery of Transcription Exercises 5.9 and 5.10 is obtained and you have studied flash cards 34 and 35, transcribe the following eight words, including one nonsense item.

1. ________	2. ________
3. ________	4. ________
5. ________	6. ________
7. ________	8. ________

Answers

'gʊdnɪs	'luk
'lʊk	'hʊp
'hup	'rʊf
'ruf	ʒu'gʊdə

The Diphthong /ɔ͜ɪ/ as in *Boy*

The /ɔ͜ɪ/ is yet another diphthong to be considered. In some other transcription systems, /o͜y/, /o͜j/, /ɔ͜y/, or /ɔ͜j/ are used. The *oy-* in *oyster* and the *-oi-* in *poignant* cover just about all the common spellings for this sound. The variations that occur in Eastern American and Southern American dialects will be discussed in Part II, Section 10 of this workbook. Do not forget to use the slur (‿) to connect the two symbols.

Transcription Exercise 5.11. Transcribing /ɔ͜ɪ/

Use this diphthong in the words that follow even if you use another sound in your dialect. Then practice saying the words. If necessary, you may confirm your transcriptions of the first three words in each column by turning to Appendix B of this workbook.

point ______________	boy ______________
destroy ______________	employ ______________
alloy ______________	Roy ______________
noise ______________	oink ______________
soy ______________	tow ______________
voice ______________	annoy ______________
loin ______________	avoid ______________

The /a͜ɪ/ Diphthong as in *High*

The /a͜ɪ/ is another common diphthong in English, but unlike the other diphthongs, its spelling patterns are slightly more ambiguous. The letter *i* is often used to represent this sound in words such as *kind* and *hide*. Do not forget to put the cap on the /a/. Dialect differences occur for this diphthong (see Transcription Exercise 5.14).

Transcription Exercise 5.12. Transcribing /a͜ɪ/

Transcribe these words using /a͜ɪ/ where applicable. Use this diphthong even if your dialect is at variance. Then practice producing it. Check your transcriptions for the first three words in each column in Appendix B of this workbook, paying special attention to the written form of this diphthong.

I ______________	sky ______________
kind ______________	buy ______________
mine ______________	ride ______________
imply ______________	employ ______________
sigh ______________	soy ______________
fight ______________	fate ______________
guide ______________	side ______________
die ______________	ironic ______________
arrive ______________	write ______________
heighten ______________	decide ______________
beside ______________	island ______________
white ______________	describe ______________
like ______________	lake ______________

Audio-Activity 5.9. Practicing Diphthongs (CD 2, Track 14)

Study flash cards 39 and 41 and complete Transcription Exercises 5.11 and 5.12. Then transcribe the following six items, including a few nonsense words. As always, check your answers with those provided.

			Answers	
1. ________	2. ________		ə'nɔ͜ɪ	dɪ'sa͜ɪd
3. ________	4. ________		'ɔ͜ɪpla͜ɪʃt	'sma͜ɪl ~ ᵊl
5. ________	6. ________		'nɔ͜ɪz̥	bla͜ɪ'plɔ͜ɪ

The Schwa Before /l/, as in *Oil*

When /l/ follows diphthongs, tense vowels, and /r/ (including the r-colored vowels), an intrusive schwa-glide often precedes the /l/. The glide is transcribed with a raised schwa (/ᵊ/). For example, *smile* may be pronounced as /'sma͜ɪl/ or /'sma͜ɪᵊl /, and *ruled* may be either /'ruld/ or /'ruᵊld/. When /l/ begins a syllable, however, the schwa-glide is less likely to occur. In *smiling*, because the /l/ begins the second syllable, the schwa-glide may not occur: /'sma͜ɪlɪŋ/.

Transcription Exercise 5.13. Practice Transcribing the Intrusive Schwa-Glide

Transcribe the following words with the schwa-glide after diphthongs and tense vowels wherever appropriate. Check your transcription of the first four items in each column by turning to Appendix B in this workbook.

wail________________	pearl________________
mild________________	pool________________
girl________________	coiled________________
talc________________	boiling________________
guile________________	hull________________
Lyle________________	gnarl________________
school________________	spoil________________
doily________________	still________________
Carl________________	stale________________
spoiling________________	smile________________

Southern American Dialect and /a͜ɪ/

In Southern American dialect, there is a tendency to remove the diphthongal aspect from /a͜ɪ/, so that either /a/ (a low-front vowel) or /ɑ/ (a low-back vowel) is used. Sometimes /æ/ might also be heard for this diphthong among some speakers of Southern American dialect.

Transcription Exercise 5.14. Dialect Variation and /a͜ɪ/

Transcribe the following into General American, and then into Southern American dialect, using /a/ (use the /a/ symbol instead of /ɑ/, for practice). The first two words are transcribed in Appendix B of this workbook.

General American	**Southern American /a/**
I________________	________________
wise________________	________________
Bible________________	________________

island______________________ ______________________________

ice cubes____________________ ______________________________

Audio-Activity 5.10. Listening for Dialect Variations (CD 2, Track 15)

When you have successfully completed Transcription Exercise 5.14 and checked flash card 43 for the correct phonetic symbol, you will be ready to listen to these pairs of words as may be pronounced in both General American or Southern American dialects. Transcribe these six items as appropriate.

		Answers	
1. ______	2. ______	ˈpra͜ɪz̥	ˈpraz̥
3. ______	4. ______	ˈtrat	ˈtra͜ɪt
5. ______	6. ______	ˈfa͜ɪn ˌra͜ɪs	ˈfan ˌras

Transcription Exercise 5.15. Transcription Review

Transcribe the following words and short phrases using your own dialect as a reference. Do not forget to show vowel reduction where necessary. Also watch your use of the primary stress marker, syllabics, the slur under diphthongs, caps on the symbols used for some of the diphthongs, and the general rules for devoicing of final-position /z̥/. Should your own dialect be at variance with the sounds covered in this section and you lack a symbol because it has not been introduced yet, then be guided by the procedures outlined for transcription in this section. It is important to learn to perceive and produce sounds, even if we do not always use them in our own speech.

dustpans______________________	passerby______________________
gorillas______________________	exercise______________________
rivals______________________	bottles______________________
shotgun______________________	sign posts______________________
principle______________________	hoi poiloi______________________
drippings______________________	bookshops______________________
once______________________	crackers______________________
days______________________	pointless______________________
constitute______________________	shrunk______________________
ballad______________________	renegade______________________
ambassador______________________	aggravate______________________
pirate ships______________________	drinkable______________________
foiled______________________	attendance______________________
unmodified______________________	stepladders______________________
visual______________________	princes______________________
dishes______________________	ambrosia______________________
fly______________________	boyhood______________________
separation______________________	aversion______________________
flanked______________________	gracious______________________
Prussia______________________	motivates______________________
fireplace______________________	valentine______________________
vitamin______________________	grapevine______________________

Audio-Activity 5.11. Auditory Review (CD 2, Track 16)

Transcribe these eight words taken from Transcription Exercise 5.15. Use the principles taught in this and previous sections of this workbook. Check your answers, if necessary.

1. ________ 2. ________
3. ________ 4. ________
5. ________ 6. ________
7. ________ 8. ________

Answers

'væləntа͜ɪn	'prinᵗsəpl̩
'pɔ͜ɪnˀlɪs	æ'bæsəɾɚ̂
'prʌʃə	'va͜ɪt̬əmən
'prɪnᵗsəz̥	'greʃəs

Transcription Exercise 5.16. Optional Advanced Transcription

The words in this exercise contain some of the sounds that will be introduced in Section 6.

throughout________________	couch________________
university________________	chimpanzee ________________
lunchroom________________	approachable________________
adjutant________________	Norwegian________________
principle ________________	awning ________________
prearrange________________	pauper________________
romance________________	feathery________________
withdraw________________	weatherproof________________
sixteenth________________	principalship________________
lethargy________________	swarthier________________

SECTION 6

Consonants: /θ, ð, tʃ, dʒ/
Vowels and Diphthong: /i, ɔ, a͜ʊ/

Learning Activities: An Introduction to the Sounds in Section 6

Learning Activity 6.1. More Vowels: /i, ɔ, a͜ʊ/

Read about these sounds in Chapters 10 (p. 217), 12 (p. 287), and 13 (p. 308) of *Applied Phonetics (AP)*. Then write the phonetic symbol that best fits each description.

1. The highest of the front vowels: ______
2. The low-front-to-high-back diphthong: ______
3. The “open o”: ______
4. Of these sounds, which is the most affected by dialect? ______
5. The mid-back lax vowel: ______
6. Of these sounds, which may occur in word-final position? ______

Learning Activity 6.2. More Fricatives and the Affricates: /θ, ð/ *and* /tʃ, dʒ/

Read about these sounds in Chapters 6 (pp. 119–129) and 7 (pp. 156–168) in *AP*. Then answer the following questions.

1. What is a fricative? ______
   ______
2. What is an affricate? ______
3. What is the symbol for the voiced interdental fricative? ______
4. What is the symbol for the voiceless alveopalatal affricate? ______
5. What is the symbol for the theta? ______
6. What is the symbol for the voiceless interdental fricative? ______
7. What is the symbol for the voiced alveopalatal affricate? ______
8. What is the symbol of for the eth? ______

Working with the Distinctive Features

A knowledge of distinctive feature theory (as in Chomsky & Halle, 1968) is necessary for the student of phonetics. When accounting for changes in pronunciation, historical or otherwise, distinctive features can be of great assistance. The purpose of these learning activities is to demonstrate how distinctive features may be used to account for sound changes. You will need to refer to the distinctive feature chart in *AP*, page 40.

Learning Activity 6.3. Comparing the Distinctive Features for the Stop Consonants

Review the material in Chapters 3 (p. 35) and 4 (pp. 47–51) in *AP* on Distinctive Features (Chomsky & Halle, 1968). Then turn to each of the stop consonants in Chapter 5 (Division 7) and become familiar with the features for each sound. (Refer to pages) Then complete the partial list of features by putting in the pluses and minuses for the stops. The first two features are done for you. Note especially the features for /t/ because we will use them in Learning Activity 6.5.

/p/	/b/	/t/	/d/	/k/	/g/
−Vocalic	−Vocalic	−Vocalic	−Vocalic	−Vocalic	−Vocalic
+Consonantal	+Consonantal	+Consonantal	+Consonantal	+Consonantal	+Consonantal
Coronal	Coronal	Coronal	Coronal	Coronal	Coronal
Anterior	Anterior	Anterior	Anterior	Anterior	Anterior
High	High	High	High	High	High
Back	Back	Back	Back	Back	Back
Voiced	Voiced	Voiced	Voiced	Voiced	Voiced

Now answer these questions based on the distinctive feature matrix that you have produced.

1. Which feature separates /p/ and /b/? ________________
2. Which feature do /b/ and /g/ share that /d/ does not have? ________________
3. Which three features separate /p/ and /k/?________________
4. What sound does /t/ become if we change the +Coronal feature to −Coronal? ________________

Learning Activity 6.4. Analyzing More Sounds Using Distinctive Features

As before, refer to the distinctive feature charts in *AP* (pp. 39, 40) before answering these questions.

1. Examine the distinctive features for each of the nasals. Which nasal is +Coronal? ________________
2. Is it the nasals or the stops that have the distinctive feature +Sonorant? ________________
3. Which is the only nasal that has the distinctive feature +High? ________________
4. /l/ and /r/ differ from each other on four distinctive features. These are: ________________
5. In the sounds /i/, /ɔ/, and /aʊ/, which is the only one that carries the distinctive feature +Tense?____
6. In the sounds /i/, /ɔ/, and /a͜ʊ/, which is the only sound that changes from −Round to +Round during its production? ________________
7. In the sounds /θ/, /ð/, /tʃ/, and /dʒ/, which two sounds have the distinctive feature +Distributed? ______
8. Which is the only distinctive feature that distinguishes /θ/ from /f/ and /s/? ________________
9. Which four features distinguish /v/ and /p/?________________
10. Which two features distinguish /ʃ/ and /dʒ/?________________
11. Which two features distinguish /s/ and /ʃ/? ________________
12. Which features distinguish /i/ and /ŋ/? ________________

Learning Activity 6.5. Working with a Familiar Phonological Rule

In Section 3 of this book (Transcription Exercise 3.1) you learned that intervocalic /t/ becomes /t̬/. In Chapter 4 of *AP* ("Reading and Writing Phonological Rules with Distinctive Features"), a rule for this sound change was explained. The rule stated that a stop consonant that is −Voiced and +Coronal will be pronounced as a stop consonant that is +Voiced and +Coronal when it occurs between vowels, if the vowel following is −Stress. In other words, /t/ will be pronounced like /d/ when it occurs between a vowel and an unstressed vowel. If this explanation is not sufficient, then read the complete explanation in *AP* (pp. 49–51)

Using this phonological rule, transcribe the following words, first phonemically (broad transcription) and then according to the rule. If the rule does not apply, then write the feature part of the rule that is violated in the space provided. The first two words are done for you.

	Broad Transcription	**Rule Applied (with Diacritic)**
better	bɛtɚ	bɛt̬ɚ
ladder	lædɚ	+Voiced
letter		
packer		
pepper		
let 'er		
matter		
clatter		
attack		
hitter		

Note: If you were to transcribe /d/ instead of /t/, others might think that you had made a serious error. In addition, you could not differentiate in your transcriptions of *latter* and *ladder*; they would both be /ˈlædɚ/. Therefore, the diacritic for voicing or partial voicing ([̬]) is used under the /t/. As you know, this diacritic is never used on a symbol for a normally voiced sound because it would be meaningless. It is acceptable practice, however, to use /d/ for ambiguous contexts, such as when you do not know if the actual word is *latter* or *ladder*, because both are pronounced alike.

Learning Activity 6.6. Distinctive Features, Syllabics, and Homorganicity

For this activity, you will need to refer to the distinctive feature chart in *AP*, page 35. Remember that in Transcription Exercise 3.4, words such as *open* and *broken* were transcribed to represent both formal and informal pronunciations. Formally, *open* is /ˈopən/; informally, /ˈopm̩/. Formally *broken* is /ˈbrokən/; informally, /ˈbrokŋ̍/. Analysis with distinctive features will illuminate the shift from formal to informal usage. It should be clear, for example, that nasals used as syllabics (/m̩, n̩, ŋ̍/) have the same set of features as nonsyllabic nasals, except for the addition of the feature +Syllabic. When the informal pronunciation is adopted, the nasal becomes +Syllabic and takes on the articulatory position of the previous stop. In other words, the nasal shares a homorganic relation with the stop.

a. When formal /ˈopən/ changes to informal /ˈopm̩/:
   1. What distinctive feature makes /m/ different from /n/? ____________________
   2. Which of these sounds (/m/ or /n/) shares this feature with /p/? ____________________
   3. Which of these three sounds are therefore homorganic? ____________________
   4. Which of these sounds becomes +Syllabic? ____________________

b. When formal /ˈbrokən/ changes to informal /ˈbrokn̩/:
1. Which four distinctive features differentiate /n/ and /ŋ/? ____________________
____
2. Which of these sounds (/n/ or /ŋ/) shares these four features with /k/? ____________________
3. Which of these three sounds are therefore homorganic? ____________________
4. Which of these sounds becomes +Syllabic? ____________________

Learning to Transcribe These Sounds: Consonants: /θ, ð, tʃ, dʒ/ Vowels and Diphthong: /i, ɔ, aʊ/

Introduction

With the study of these seven additional symbols, the basic inventory of American English sounds will be complete. You have already had some experience with three of these symbols. Two of these sounds, /tʃ/ and /dʒ/, are the result of combining symbols learned previously, and one of them, /ɔ/, was introduced before as part of the diphthong /ɔɪ/. The remaining vowel sound, /i/, is familiar from orthography, but requires learning a new sound value for it.

The /ɔ/ as in *Caught* in Some Dialects

Perhaps no sound in the English language is as influenced by dialect as is this vowel. In fact, many speakers of the language do not use it in their speech and therefore have great difficulty in learning to perceive and transcribe it. Yet no sound teaches us better the need for ear training if we are to be able to transcribe what was actually spoken rather than what we *think* was spoken.

You can approximate this sound by isolating the /l/ sound in *milk.* You will note that the tongue is low and back in the mouth for this particular /l/ sound. Once you can make this velar /l/, produce it while simultaneously rounding and protruding the lips. The result is /ɔ/.

Previously you studied the diphthong /ɔɪ/, and reference was made to its dialect variations (also see Section 10 of this workbook). We now consider those dialects in which /ɔ/ is phonemic. If you differentiate in your speech between *cot* (/kɑt/) and *caught* (/kɔt/), then you probably already have the /ɔ/ sound in your dialect. If you do not make this distinction, you will need to work especially hard on developing your ear for this sound. Although the /ɔ/ exists routinely in Eastern American and Southern American dialects, it has been replaced in other dialects by /ɑ/, or a slightly rounded low back vowel that is transcribed /ɒ/.

Some spelling conventions might aid in remembering when this sound occurs. The spelling *o* represents /ɔ/ or /ɒ/ before voiceless fricatives, /f, θ, s/, before a voiced velar stop, /g/, and before the velar nasal, /ŋ/, as in *off, moth, boss, fog*, and *thong*. Otherwise, orthographic *o* is usually pronounced /ɑ/. In parts of New England, whenever it does not represent the tense vowel /o/, the spelling *o* represents /ə/ or /ɒ/, as in *optimum*. The spellings *au*, *aw* and *al* usually represent this sound, as in *haul, saw*. and *all*. Less frequent spellings for this sound are *augh* in *caught*, *ough* in *thought*, and *wa-* or *war* in *want, wash, water*, and *warden*.

Transcription Exercise 6.1. Transcribing /ɔ/

Use /ɔ/, even if you lack this sound in your dialect. Learn to use the spelling conventions just described. Then, practice producing this sound. Note that some words are included that *do not* contain the /ɔ/ sound. In case this sound is a problem for you, you may check your transcriptions of the first four words in each column in Appendix B.

bought____________	brought____________
audible____________	vaunt____________
often____________	sprawl____________
fog____________	haul____________

anoint______	cough______
abroad______	small______
song______	taught______
wrought______	root______
log______	long ______
clause______	lisp______
salt______	loss______
lass______	call______
hog______	sought______

Audio-Activity 6.1. Listening for the Difference Between /ɑ/ and /ɔ/ (CD 2, Track 17)

In this activity, listen for the difference in pronunciation between /ɑ/, a sound that you already know, and /ɔ/, a difficult sound for those who do not have it in their dialects. Write only the phonetic symbol for /ɔ/ or /ɑ/ to represent the vowel that you hear in each of the 10 words that follow. Do not transcribe the entire word. Check your answers with those provided.

1. ______	2. ______	/ɔ/	/ɑ/
3. ______	4. ______	/ɔ/	/ɔ/
5. ______	6. ______	/ɑ/	/ɑ/
7. ______	8. ______	/ɔ/	/ɔ/
9. ______	10. ______	/ɑ/	/ɔ/

(Last two columns: **Answers**)

The Shift from /ɔ/ and /ɑ/ to /ɒ/

Wise (1957) reports that /ɒ/ is not as long in duration as /ɔ/. The lips, while still rounded, are not protruded to the extent usually required for /ɔ/. Otherwise, the two sounds are alike. Speakers who do not have /ɔ/ in their dialects may have /ɒ/. The /ɒ/ sound is really /ɑ/ or /a/, but with lip rounding. Interestingly, there appears to be a trend among speakers of American English to use /ɒ/ instead of /ɑ/ or /ɔ/.

Transcription Exercise 6.2. Transcribing Words with /ɒ/

Practice saying and transcribing /ɒ/ in these words.

got______	fought______
dog______	soft______
gone______	vault______
across ______	belong______
saw ______	cause______
frog______	pawed______

Audio-Activity 6.2. Listening for the Shift from /ɔ/ and /ɑ/ to /ɒ/ (CD 2, Track 18)

For this activity, listen carefully to the three slightly different pronunciations that you have studied in Transcription Exercises 6.1 and 6.2. In the 12 words for transcription, the first 6 are three pronunciations of two words.

			Answers	
1. _______	2. _______		ˈhɔg	ˈhɒg
3. _______	4. _______		ˈhɑg	ˈfɑt
5. _______	6. _______		ˈfɒt	ˈfɔt
7. _______	8. _______		ˈgɒt	ˈdɔg
9. _______	10. _______		ˈgɒn	ˈkɒz̥
11. _______	12. _______		ˈsɔ	ˈɑn

Contrasting /ɔ/ and /ɔ͜ɪ/ in *Lawn* and *Loin*

There is a marked difference between the way /ɔ/ is pronounced as a phoneme and as the first sound in the diphthong /ɔ͜ɪ/. Students often wonder why. One reason is that the duration of /ɔ/ is usually longer than the first part of the diphthong. Preparation for the glide to the high front space, represented by the lax /ɪ/ requires that the /ɔ/ be shortened. Another difference is that some speakers tend to begin the diphthong slightly higher than usual /ɔ/ production, approximating the /o/. The only solution to this dilemma is to learn that the International Phonetic Association (IPA) alphabet symbols happen to be /ɔ/ and /ɔ͜ɪ/, even if the similarity appears remote.

Transcription Exercise 6.3. Contrasting /ɔ/ and /ɔ͜ɪ/

Transcribe these words, using these symbols where appropriate, even if your dialect is at variance with the resulting pronunciations. The first two words in each column are transcribed in Appendix B.

boil ______________________ ball ______________________
loin ______________________ lawn ______________________
toy saw ______________________ soy ______________________
tall ______________________ toil ______________________
annoy ______________________ fried ______________________
fraud ______________________ Freud ______________________

The /ɔ/ + /r/ Combination as in *Core*

Students of phonetics often want to transcribe words such as *born* with /or/, following spelling convention, instead of /ɔr/. This might be an acceptable form for some dialects and for some transcription systems. However, our recommendation is that you learn to use /ɔr/ for the General American pronunciation. Many phoneticians transcribe /ɔr/ as /ɔ͜ɚ/. Despite its popularity, we see little advantage to this convention. Rather we recommend that /ɔ͜ɚ/ (or even /o͜ɚ/) be used to transcribe those productions made with a definite offglide, thus keeping the /ɔr/ for broad (phonemic) transcriptions. Compare /skɔr/ to /skɔ͜ɚ/ and /sko͜ɚ/. In some dialects, a difference is made between *horse* (/hɔrs/) and *hoarse* (/ho͜ɚs/). In Southern American, /hɔs/ or /ho͜ʊəs/ are common pronunciations for *horse*.

Transcription Exercise 6.4. Transcribing /ɔr/

Where applicable, use /ɔr/ even if your dialect varies from the resulting pronunciations, unless your instructor tells you otherwise. You may compare your transcriptions for the first two words in each column by looking in Appendix B of this workbook.

score ______________________ born ______________________
forward ______________________ organized ______________________

corner ____________________ poured ____________________

Norse ____________________ or ____________________

storm ____________________ warm ____________________

normal ____________________ shore ____________________

lord ____________________ mortar ____________________

The Shift from /ɔr/ to /ɑr/

In some varieties of General American dialect, and especially in Southern American, /ɔr/ may shift to /ɑr/.

Transcription Exercise 6.5. Differentiating between /ɔr/ and /ɑr/

Using your own pronunciation as a guide, transcribe the following words noting whether you use /ɔr/ or /ɑr/. Then practice the alternate pronunciation.

My Dialect	Alternate Pronunciation
foreign ____________________	____________________
Warren ____________________	____________________
moral ____________________	____________________
horrible ____________________	____________________
quarrel ____________________	____________________
tomorrow ____________________	____________________
forest ____________________	____________________
horoscope ____________________	____________________
sorrow ____________________	____________________
Oregon ____________________	____________________

Audio-Activity 6.3. Listening for Vowel + /r/ Combinations (CD 2, Track 19)

This activity is based on Transcription Exercises 6.4 and 6.5. Locate and study flash cards 45 and 46. Transcribe each of these words with /ɔr/ or /ɑr/, depending on how each is pronounced. There are six words.

1. ________ 2. ________

3. ________ 4. ________

5. ________ 6. ________

Answers

ˈsɔro	ˈmɑrl̩
ˈfɑrɪd	ˈkwɔrəl
ˈɑrəndʒ	ˈfɔrən

The Vowel /i/ as in *Bee*

It would appear that few problems would result from the transcription of this vowel once the transcriber had made the sound-symbol association. However, there are areas for variation and confusion that will now be discussed.

Transcription Exercise 6.6. Transcribing /i/

The first three words in each column are transcribed in Appendix B of this workbook. Check your transcriptions carefully because not every word requires /i/ in its transcription.

heat ____________	heed ____________
unbeatable ____________	extreme ____________
preschool ____________	speed ____________
tease ____________	system ____________
relieve ____________	teamwork ____________
leave ____________	lift ____________
machine ____________	belief ____________
Greek ____________	crease ____________
receive ____________	nonphonemic ____________

Transcribing /ɪ/ or /i/ in Word-Final Position

There is some question among phoneticians as to whether /i/ can occur in words or affixes ending with *y*, *i*, or the *-ly* combination. For example, in the word *easy*, do you say /'izi/ or /'izɪ/? If you speak a form of Southern American, the tendency would be toward /ɪ/, but other speakers may produce a sound closer to /i/. As a transcriber, you need to become aware that speakers vary. Whereas IPA tradition suggests the use of /ɪ/ in such contexts, it may well be that a particular speaker produces a sound more similar to /i/. However, that same speaker may shift toward /ɪ/ in informal or connected speech. Perhaps another phonetic symbol is needed to represent a non-tense /i/, because phonetic practice is away from using a tense vowel in weaker syllables.

Transcription Exercise 6.7. Using /i/ *or* /ɪ/ *in Word-Final Position*

Transcribe these words, using your pronunciation as a guide. Unless your instructor says otherwise, /i/ is acceptable in word-final position.

greedy ____________	believe ____________
pity ____________	continually ____________
vocabulary ____________	polysyllabic ____________
polygamy ____________	slowly ____________
polyglot ____________	valiantly ____________
yummy ____________	semiconductor ____________
Nancy ____________	company ____________
university ____________	immediately ____________
beauty ____________	beautify ____________

Audio-Activity 6.4. Listening for /i/ *(CD 2, Track 20)*

This listening activity is based on Transcription Exercises 6.6 and 6.7, emphasizing /i/. Transcribe these six words.

1. ______ 2. ______
3. ______ 4. ______
5. ______ 6. ______

Answers

rə'liv	'gridi
'bj͜ut̬ɪfa͜ɪ	'bj͜ut̬i
mə'ʃin	'nænᵗsi

Nasalization and the /ɪ/–/i/ Contrast

You might have wondered back in Section 2 why we had you transcribe *pink* with the /ɪ/ symbol instead of /i/. Many transcribers, it appears, perceive the high front vowel /i/ preceding the velar nasal /ŋ/. We have already made the observation that, in some dialects, there is a shift in pronouncing *pen* so that it is the same as *pin*. The same process of raising the vowel may also operate to cause /ɪ/ to appear as /i/ before the velar nasal in the same dialects. In addition, /æ/ may approach /e/ before the velar nasal.

What happens is that coupling the oral cavity with the nasal cavity causes these front vowels to be nasalized. This alters their quality so that they seem to be shifting in the direction of the higher vowel: /ɪ/ to /i/ and /æ/ to /e/. Some speakers have then proceeded to pronounce these as higher vowels.

The dilemma for the transcriber is to show this tendency without running the risk of having the transcription viewed as a mistake. In other words, /pɪŋk/ is always considered correct, whereas /piŋk/ is not. To overcome this problem, we recommend either using brackets [ ], showing that the transcription is narrow, or marking the vowel with the diacritic for nasalization /˜/ in the event that brackets are not used.

Transcription Exercise 6.8. Practicing /i/ Preceding /ŋ/

Transcribe in your own dialect, noting your particular pronunciation of /ɪ/ before the velar nasal /ŋ/. Do you tend to pronounce /i/? If so, do you also say /pɪn/ for both *pen* and *pin*? In those words ending in *-ing*, do you say /-ɪŋ/, /-ɪn/, /-iŋ/ or /-in/? What happens to /æ/ before /ŋ/ in your speech?

Note: If you tend to use /i/ in these items, transcribe with /ɪ/, marking it for nasalization, /ɪ̃/. Also use /æ̃/ instead of /e/ before any nasal sound in these words.

bring ________	sink ________
anchor ________	noting ________
drank ________	putting ________
resulting ________	gang ________
fingerling ________	mingle ________
slingshot ________	lingering ________
clinging ________	bullying ________
wedding ring ________	cravings ________
fang ________	Bangkok ________
satisfying ________	tingling ________

Audio-Activity 6.5. Listening for the Nasalization of /ɪ/ with /ŋ/ (CD 2, Track 21)

Remember to transcribe the tenser vowel as suggested in Transcription Exercise 6.8 with a nasalizing diacritic over /ɪ/. Transcribe these six words.

1. ________ 2. ________
3. ________ 4. ________
5. ________ 6. ________

Answers

ˈsɪ̃ŋk	ˈbrɪ̃ŋ
ˈtɪ̃ŋglɪ̃ŋ	ˈmɪ̃ŋgl̩
ˈnot̬ɪ̃ŋ	bʊliɪ̃ŋ

Transcribing /ɪr/ or /ir/

Still another difficulty that students of phonetics often have is that of making their pronunciations jibe with a longstanding tradition among American phoneticians: the use of /ɪr/ when their perceptions dictate the use of /ir/. This convention may have been the result of generalizing from Southern American dialect in which *fear* is pronounced /fɪr/, or even /fɪ͜ə/. Other speakers use a pronunciation that is closer to /fir/. Once again, we recommend that the student learn to perceive and transcribe *both* pronunciations. We do, however, recommend the use of /ir/ as an acceptable transcription for this combination. We also recommend that the use of /ɪ͜ɚ/ or /i͜ɚ/ be reserved for productions spoken with a definite offglide, as clearly seen in the words *barrier* and *carrier*.

Transcription Exercise 6.9. Transcribing /i/ *or* /ɪ/ *Preceding* /r/

Be consistent in your transcriptions of these words. Listen for alternate pronunciations in the speech of those around you.

rear ________	appear ________
experience ________	merely ________
material ________	spirit ________
hurried ________	irrigation ________
smear ________	soar ________
irritate ________	beard ________
seriously ________	year ________
fearful ________	cashier ________

Audio-Activity 6.6. Listening for the Difference Between /ir/ *and* /ɪr/ *(CD 2, Track 22)*

Locate and study flash card 47. Transcribe these seven words according to their pronunciations. Also, be prepared to transcribe two syllables with one of these vowels plus schwar in words 4 and 7.

1. ______	2. ______
3. ______	4. ______
5. ______	6. ______
7. ______	

Answers

ˈsiriz	ˈfɪrfl̩
ˈspɪrɪt	ˈmɛriɚ
əˈpir	məˈtɪrɪəl
ˈhæpiɚ	

The Diphthong /a͜ʊ/ as in *How*

Once again, the transcriber must remember to cap both symbols that comprise this diphthong, and connect both symbols with a slur below. There are few problems in the broad transcription of this sound. As your ability to transcribe becomes more refined, you will want to attend to the variations that occur in the onset portion of this diphthong as discussed in *AP* (see page 308).

Transcription Exercise 6.10. Transcribing /a͜ʊ/

Transcribe these words carefully because not every one requires this diphthong in its transcription. Also review the schwa-glide in Transcription Exercise 5.13. Check your transcriptions for the first three words in each column by turning to Appendix B.

cloud ________	amounts ________
town ________	cow ________
flounder____ ________	sauerkraut ________
growled ________	howling ________
outer space ________	shout ________

pound ____________	pond ____________
powder____________	groaned____________
sounds____________	vowel____________
house____________	ground____________
doubt____________	short ____________

Audio-Activity 6.7. Listening for the /a͜ʊ/ Diphthong (CD 2, Track 23)

Before completing this listening activity, study flash card 40. There are six words containing this diphthong.

1. ______ 2. ______

3. ______ 4. ______

5. ______ 6. ______

Answers

ˈsa͜ʊnz̥	əˈma͜ʊnts
ˈma͜ʊnʔn̩	ˈna͜ʊ
ˈgra͜ʊnd	ˈpa͜ʊnd

The Consonants /θ/ as in *Thigh* and /ð/ as in *Thy*

The first task for the transcriber is to learn that /θ/ is voiceless and /ð/ is voiced. Otherwise, the production of these sounds is very similar. Because these sounds, especially /θ/, tend to be weakly made, the student often has difficulty discerning exactly when the sound is voiced or voiceless. Perhaps a few generalizations will help.

1. In the initial position, /θ/ occurs in all content words and /ð/ occurs in all function words except *through*. Therefore, /ð/ begins these very common words: *the, this/that, these/those, they/their/them, then, there, than, though.*
2. In word-medial position (between vowels) /ð/ is used for nonforeign words. Therefore, /ð/ is used in *mother* and *father*, but not for *ether* that is of Greek origin.
3. In word-final position, when the word is a noun, /θ/ is used; but when the word is a verb, /ð/ occurs. Compare *bath* and *bathe*, and *teeth* and *teethe*. Interestingly enough, this same tendency is found for the other fricatives. When a voiceless fricative ends a word, that word will more than likely be a noun, but when a verb, a voiced fricative will be used. Compare *grass* and *graze* and *use* (noun) and *use* (verb).
4. Finally, be sure to maintain the voiced/voiceless feature across *both* sounds in blends so that plurals, for example, will be transcribed /ðz/ and /θs/ in *bathes* and *baths*.

Transcription Exercise 6.11. Transcribing /θ/ and /ð/

The first two words in each column are transcribed in Appendix B.

there____________	thus____________
theft____________	thirst ____________
thousand ____________	thyself____________
bother ____________	thumbtack____________
thermometer____________	fatherly ____________
cloth____________	clothe____________
clothing____________	breathe ____________
breathing____________	breath____________

booths ____________	zenith ____________
orthodox ____________	nevertheless ____________
north ____________	northern ____________
orthography ____________	aesthetic ____________
weather ____________	Thursday ____________
hypothesis ____________	toothpaste ____________

Audio-Activity 6.8. Listening for the Interdental Fricatives (CD 2, Track 24)

These sounds are found on flash cards 9 and 10. Transcribe these 10 items, some of which are nonsense words.

1. ______	2. ______
3. ______	4. ______
5. ______	6. ______
7. ______	8. ______
9. ______	10. ______

Answers

ˈθɛft	ˈðaɪ̯
ˈnɔrðɚn	ˈðip
ˈsið	ˈmiθən
ˈθaɪ̯	ˈðuʃən
ˈbɑðɚ	ˈθɪftɚ

Additional Practice With the Voiced/Voiceless Distinction

advice ____________	advise ____________
refuse (noun) ____________	refuse (verb) ____________
loose (adj.) ____________	lose (verb) ____________
safe ____________	save ____________
half ____________	halve ____________
life ____________	live (verb) ____________
lath ____________	lathe ____________
sheath ____________	sheathe ____________

The Affricates: /tʃ/ as in *Chip* and /dʒ/ as in *Gyp*

The affricates are sounds that change their manner of articulation during their production. They begin with a stop and end with a fricative. Instead of releasing the /t/ and /d/ stops with aspiration, they are released with fricative turbulence. The /tʃ/ is voiceless, and the /dʒ/ is voiced. Due to your previous experience with /t/ and /d/ as stops and the /ʃ/ and /ʒ/ as fricatives, the task of making this sound-symbol association should not be difficult. The letters *ch* or *tch* usually represent the /tʃ/, as in *church* and *watch*. For /dʒ/, the letters *g* and *j* are often used, as in *George* and *Jack*. One very common convention is to transcribe these sounds with the c-wedge (or c-check), written /č/, for /tʃ/ and the j-wedge (or j-check), written /ǰ/, for /dʒ/. In the exercises that follow, use /tʃ/ and /dʒ/ unless told differently by your instructor.

Transcription Exercise 6.12. The Affricates

Transcribe these words in your own speech. The first three words in each column are transcribed in Appendix B should you need to review your transcriptions before completing the exercise.

chime ______	church ______
gent ______	jinx ______
jammed ______	chamber ______
future ______	generation ______
educate ______	origin ______
hitchhike ______	culture ______
teaching ______	indigestible ______
leather jacket ______	cheesecloth ______
angelfish ______	injurious ______
childbirth ______	conjecture ______
perpetuate ______	researched ______
garbage ______	endangered ______
surcharge ______	majority ______
archbishop ______	changed ______

Audio-Activity 6.9. Listening for the Affricates (CD 2, Track 25)

Study flash cards 16 and 17 and then transcribe these eight words that contain the affricate sounds. Check your answers with those provided if necessary.

1. ______	2. ______
3. ______	4. ______
5. ______	6. ______
7. ______	8. ______

Answers

ˈsɝdʒ	ˈkʌltʃɚ
ˈɪndʒɚi	ˈdʒoks
ˈtʃendʒd	ˈlɛdʒ
ˈfju͜tʃɚ	ˈwɪtʃ

Transcribing /ʊr/, as in *Poor*

The last of the vowel + /r/ combinations to be considered is /ʊr/. In addition to the usual Southern American r-dropping differences in pronunciation, there is also considerable variation among speakers of American English for /ʊr/. Some typically use /ɔr/, as in /ˈpɔr/. Such speakers do not differentiate in their speech between the words *poor* and *pour*. Other speakers use a pronunciation closer to /ɝ/, as when *pure* (/ˈpjɔr/) is pronounced /ˈpjɝ/. When /u/ replaces /ʊ/ in this vowel + /r/ combination, the pronunciation is /u͜ɚ/, as when *poor* is said /ˈpu͜ɚ/. Common spellings for /ʊr/ are *our* as in *tour*, *ure* as in *sure*, and *oor* as in *poor*.

Transcription Exercise 6.13. Practice with /ʊr/

Transcribe these words using /ʊr/ where appropriate. If your pronunciation varies, you might want to transcribe both forms.

lure ______	spoor ______
poor ______	boor ______
sure ______	rural ______
allure ______	bureau ______

Europe ______	during ______
tour ______	your ______
pure ______	cure ______

Additional Practice with Vowel + /r/ Combinations

You have studied how certain vowels combine with /r/ to produce frequently used sequences in American English: /ɑr/, /ɛr/, /ɔr/, and /ʊr/. In words written with *ure* or *our*, especially following voiceless stops, there is some variation, even within the same speaker. Recall that words like *purify, touring*, and *cure* may be pronounced with /ɔr/, /ʊr/, and /ɝ/.

Transcription Exercise 6.14. Transcribing Vowel + /r/ Combinations

Transcribe in your own dialect.

arid ______	fearing ______
berry ______	married ______
herald ______	parents ______
forest ______	moral ______
harrow ______	corrode ______
steering ______	tourist ______
caramel ______	mulberry ______
paraffin ______	purify ______
touring ______	oriental ______
starry ______	weary ______
sorrowful ______	parroting ______
during ______	Gary ______
forum ______	jury ______
arrow ______	buried ______
cherish ______	marigold ______

Audio-Activity 6.10. Listening for Vowel + /r/ Combinations (CD 2, Track 26)

Complete Transcription Exercise 6.14 and review flash cards 45, 46, 47, and 48. Then transcribe these 10 words the way they are pronounced, especially noting the vowels before /r/.

1. ______	2. ______
3. ______	4. ______
5. ______	6. ______
7. ______	8. ______
9. ______	10. ______

Answers

ˈfɔrəm	ˈmɑrl̩
ˈstirɪŋ	ˈmæro
ˈtʃɛri	ˈfɑrəst
ˈmɔrl̩	ˈfirfl̩
ˈstɑri	ˈbæri

Transcription Exercise 6.15. Review

Transcribe using your own speech as a guide

dredged ________	windshield ________
seventh ________	old-fashioned ________
glacier ________	therefore ________
both ________	smuggling ________
smash up ________	themselves ________
mouthing ________	tunesmith ________
territory ________	sanctuary ________
sphere ________	Uruguay ________
vivacious ________	thoughtless ________
innocence ________	washcloth ________
vestibule ________	toothpaste ________
heather ________	teething ________
pathology ________	strengthen ________
should and could ________	cloudy ________
ground wire ________	snake charmer ________
tragic accident ________	crucify ________
freezing point ________	organization ________
both ________	bother ________
museum ________	Asiatic flu ________
sabotage ________	appraisal ________
thatch ________	featherstitch ________
conversion ________	retirement ________
chisel ________	triumph ________
overburdensome ________	division ________
restriction ________	originate ________
gratifying ________	seizure ________
shortsightedness ________	laundry ________
macaw ________	ringleader ________

Audio-Activity 6.11. Auditory Review (CD 2, Track 27)

This activity is based on Transcription Exercise 6.15, which reviews a number of transcription principles. Transcribe these 12 words as spoken.

1. ________	2. ________
3. ________	4. ________
5. ________	6. ________
7. ________	8. ________
9. ________	10. ________
11. ________	12. ________

Answers

ˈboθ	ˈgleʃɚ
ˈsɛvənθ	ˈtʃɪzl̩
ˈsiʒɚ	ˈθætʃ
ˈtiðĩŋ	ˈklaʊ̯di
ˈðɛrfɔr	məˈkɔ
ˈsfɪr	ˈbɑðɚ

SECTION 7

Stress in American English

Transcribers usually have little difficulty in mastering the symbols that comprise the phonetic alphabet and the sound-symbol associations necessary for using those symbols correctly. However, stress perception, even the placement of the primary stress marker, not to mention the perception of other levels of stress, presents the biggest challenge to students of phonetics. In short, you are not alone if the perception of stress is stressful for you! Yet the situation is not as bleak as you might imagine. With a slightly simplified approach to stress and its perception, you might make greater gains than you thought possible. For a more comprehensive discussion of stress, see Chapter 14 in *Applied Phonetics (AP)*.

American English stress is complicated because it is the result of a combination of factors. Nevertheless, it is primarily the result of a pitch jump (an upward pitch step) on the prominent syllable of a word, or a jump in pitch on the prominent syllable of the important word in a phrase or shorter sentence (Stern, 1987). Longer sentences may have more than one pitch jump. Look, for example, at the first word in the following exercise—*abdomen*. There are two ways to pronounce this word, one with the pitch jump on the first syllable, "AB-do-men," and the other with the pitch jump on the second syllable, "ab-DO-men." Although it is true that loudness or duration may also be used to show this prominence, pitch is used more frequently in American English, whereas loudness and duration are important to secondary stress.

The pitch jump is tied to meaning, and thus may occur in several places within an utterance. However, the English language places constraints on what happens after the pitch jump. We are required to step down in pitch on each syllable and fall in pitch on the last syllable of the word, phrase, or sentence. What this means is that primary stress occurs on the pitch jump with as many levels of secondary stress or non-stress as there are syllables in the word, phrase, or sentence. The pitch jump, then, is the main test for primary stress with secondary or non-stress relegated to the levels of pitch surrounding this high pitch point.

Practice saying these phrases and sentences as they are diagrammed. For the phrases and sentences only one possibility is given for each.

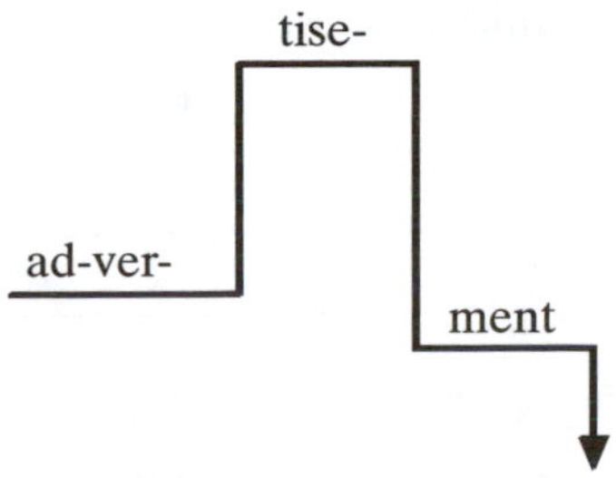

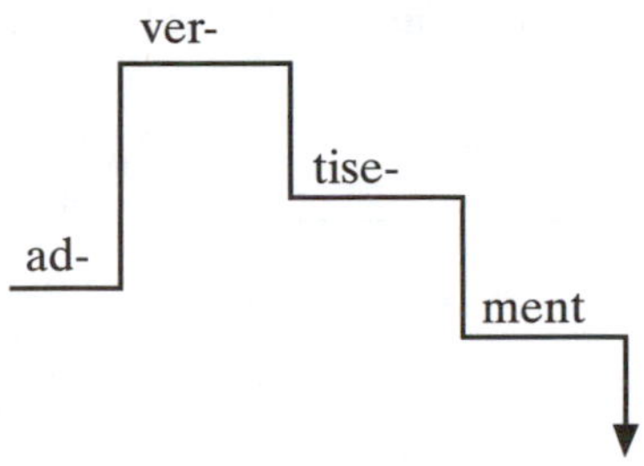

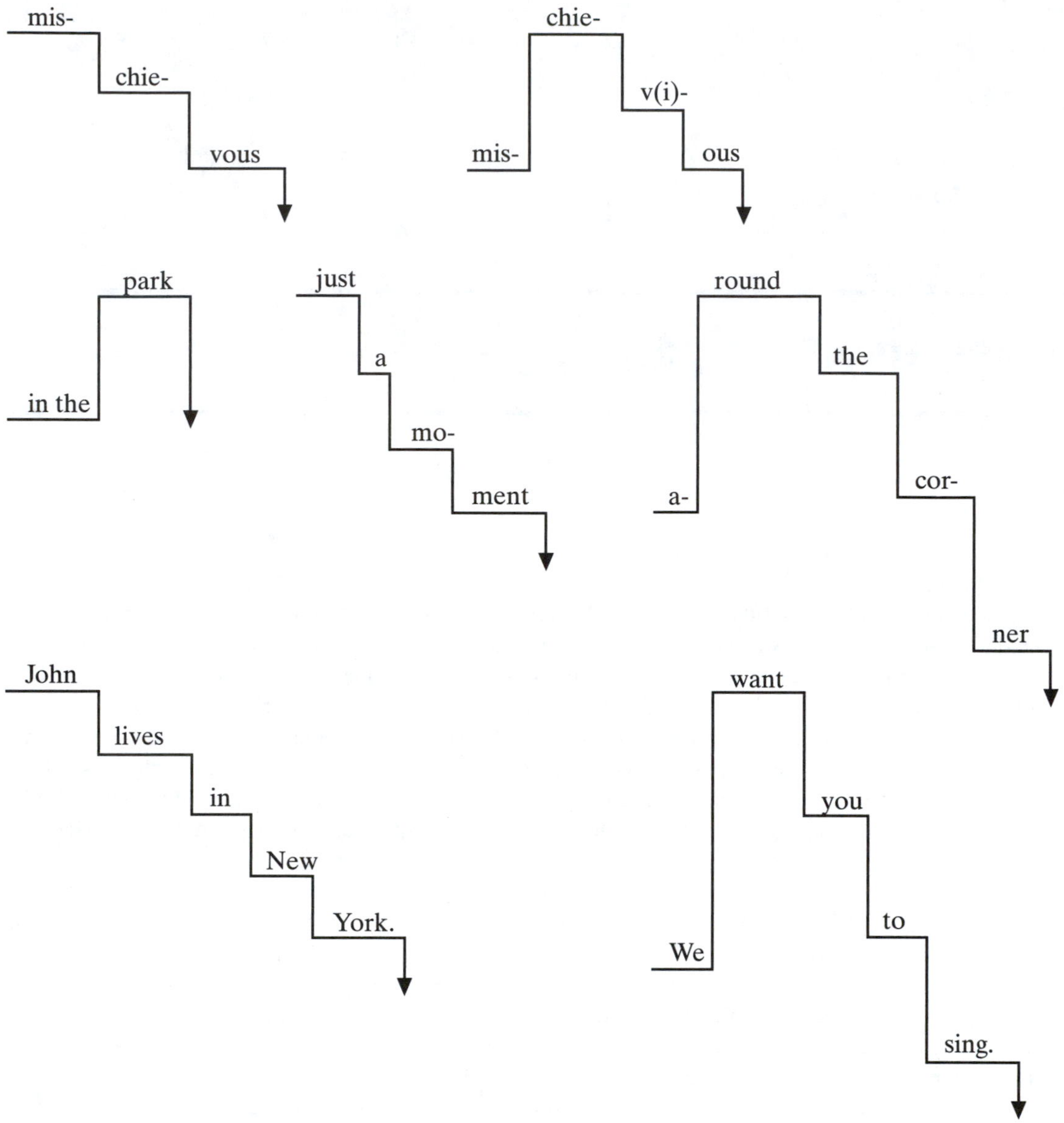

These few examples will give you the idea that American English relies heavily for its stress on pitch and that pitch is tied to particular syllables. The high pitch point is related to primary stress while other syllables are on different pitch levels.

In the exercises that follow, use the pitch test for determining where the primary stress occurs.

Transcription Exercise 7.1. Words Having Primary Stress on the First Syllable

In each of these words the primary stress marker will be placed on the first syllable. Listen to each word as you pronounce it and use the pitch test to confirm your perception of primary stress.

privacy________________	vagabond________________
calendar________________	hemisphere________________
mechanized________________	laminated________________
mannequin________________	bakery________________
changeable________________	calculate________________

Transcription Exercise 7.2. Words Having Primary Stress on the Second Syllable

Each of these words will receive the primary stress marker on the second syllable. As before, listen to your pronunciation of each word as you practice the pitch test for stress placement.

eclipse ________	producer ________
incapable ________	rambunctious ________
impress ________	maneuver ________
longevity ________	bronchitis ________
avenger ________	rehearsal ________

Transcription Exercise 7.3. Words Having Primary Stress on the Next to the Last Syllable

Many words that end with *-tion* (or *-sion* and *-cian*) and *-ic* will usually receive primary stress on the syllable that precedes the suffix. Transcribe these words, marking primary stress as fits this rule.

situation ________	patriotic ________
intermission ________	specific ________
ventilation ________	epidemic ________
education ________	terrific ________
introduction ________	supersonic ________
generation ________	mathematics ________

Transcription Exercise 7.4. Deciding on Primary Stress in Words

Now that you have been transcribing words with predictable syllable stress, it is time to test your skill. First, determine which syllable receives primary stress in the following words (first, second, or next to the last); then transcribe each using your pronunciation as a guide. The first three items in each column are transcribed in Appendix B so that you may check your work.

Canadian ________	introduction ________
principle ________	optimistic ________
embarrassment ________	syllable ________
conscious ________	supersonic ________
renewal ________	gentlemanly ________
liberty ________	mahogany ________
substantially ________	propriety ________
tamper ________	river ________
entanglement ________	rehabilitation ________

Transcription Exercise 7.5. Primary Stress in Short Phrases

A word spoken in isolation receives primary stress, even if it is only one syllable long. In fact, every word carries primary stress on some syllable if spoken alone. However, when words are used in phrases usually only one word (or syllable) is spoken with primary stress. In transcribing the items that follow, mark primary stress—one in each phrase. Remember that the caret (/ʌ/) and the reversed-hooked epsilon (/ɝ/) only occur in syllables of primary stress—syllables that have the pitch jump. The first three items in each column are transcribed in Appendix B so that you may check your work.

the__________	the book__________
a__________	a lot__________
in__________	in the park__________
a rabbit__________	the class__________
in fact__________	to glide__________
an edict__________	the robot__________
at school__________	in the water__________
to Tacoma__________	the table__________
from Washington__________	by the prison__________
on the table__________	his resignation__________

Audio-Activity 7.1. Listening for Primary Stress (CD 2, Track 28)

In this activity, listen for the syllable with the pitch jump. Then transcribe these eight words and phrases, marking the syllable on which there is a pitch jump with a primary stress.

1. ______ 2. ______
3. ______ 4. ______
5. ______ 6. ______
7. ______ 8. ______

Answers

ərə'kun	ðəwɚd'ðʌ
mə'hɑgəni	ɑn ðə 'tebl̩
tə rə'dus	aʊ̯t̬ əv 'kæ̃nədə
ɛni kə'nediən	træn'skrɪpʃənəli

Audio-Activity 7.2. Listening to Words Differing in Stress (CD 2, Track 29)

Here are some pairs of words that differ in primary stress (and also in the occurrence of reduced vowels). Some of these have different meanings; others are simply variant pronunciations of the same word. Transcribe each of these eight words being sure to mark primary stress.

1. ______ 2. ______
3. ______ 4. ______
5. ______ 6. ______
7. ______ 8. ______

Answers

'pɝmɪt	pɚ'mɪt
ə'dʌlt	'ædəlt
hɛrəsmɛnt	hə'ræsmɛnt
kən'vɝt	'kɑnvɚt

Transcription Exercise 7.6. Parts of Speech and Primary Stress

For some words that can be used either as a noun or a verb (or an adjective), the stress placement changes as the part of speech changes. Transcribe the following, using correct primary stress placement. There are some words that can change from a noun to a verb where a stress shift does not occur, for example, *consent*.

an addict__________	addicted__________
the convert__________	to convert__________
an upset__________	to upset__________
his consent__________	to consent__________
a rebel__________	to rebel__________
an extract__________	to extract__________
my delight__________	to delight__________
this permit__________	permitted__________

Transcription Exercise 7.7. Transcribing Alternate Pronunciations

The following words have alternate pronunciations in American English. Some are pronounced with a shift in primary stress from one syllable to another, whereas others are spoken with different sounds, but no change in stress. Transcribe each word into your own pronunciation, then check your pronunciation with that of your fellow students to see if yours is the majority one (the pronunciation used by most of your friends). Use the pitch test to determine the syllable of primary stress. Mark it appropriately. The asterisks will become important as you do Exercise 7.8.

*abdomen________________	apricot________________
height________________	*zoology________________
neither________________	*interesting________________
*harassment________________	comparable________________
advertisement________________	bouquet________________
coupon________________	finance________________
adult________________	forehead________________
homage________________	*insurance________________
mischievous________________	often________________
humble________________	illustrative________________

Transcription Exercise 7.8. The Pitch Test

Apply the pitch test to the five words marked with an asterisk (*) in Transcription Exercise 7.7. Diagram your pronunciation for each word.

Example:

Marking Secondary Stress in Multisyllabic Words

As we will see in Section 9, assigning secondary stress is important in transcribing connected speech. For transcribing multisyllabic words, it may also be used. In a word like *colony*, /ˈkɑləni/, there is only one stressed syllable; in *colonization*, /kɑlənɪˈzeʃən/, there are two stressed syllables, one of them weaker than the other. The pitch test will result in this diagram:

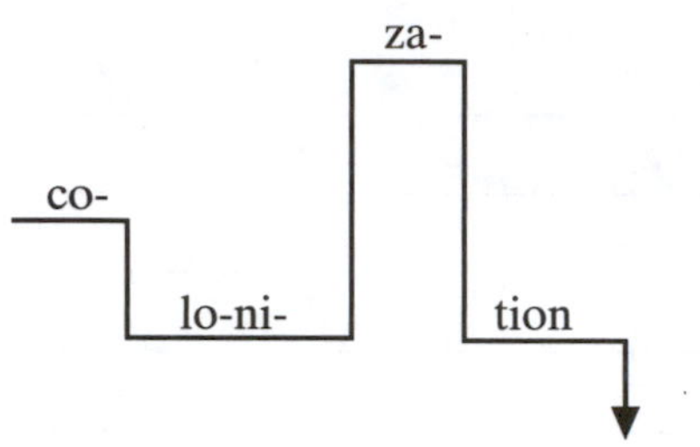

Transcription Exercise 7.9. Two Levels of Stress in Words

Transcribe these items, indicating two levels of stress where appropriate. Check your transcription of the first two items in each column in Appendix B.

Note: In some transcription systems, the caret /ʌ/ and reversed, hooked epsilon /ɝ/ may be used in syllables that receive either primary or secondary stress. For pedagogical purposes, we have opted to use these symbols only in syllables that receive primary stress to avoid some of the problems in trying to decide whether a particular speaker has intended secondary or nonstress.

anthropology______________________
apologetic______________________
delicatessen______________________
consideration______________________
sociology______________________
Oklahoma______________________
exaggeration______________________
dilapidated______________________
embryonic______________________
nationality______________________
biographic______________________
radioactive______________________

Transcription Exercise 7.10. Word Sets Differing in Stress

Transcribe these related sets of words, noticing what changes in primary and secondary stress occur as word class changes.

telegraph______________________
telegraphic______________________
integrity______________________
separation______________________
indent______________________
microscope______________________
origin______________________
originate______________________
compete______________________
confide______________________
tolerance______________________
personal______________________
telegraphy______________________
integral______________________
integration______________________
separatist______________________
indentation______________________
microscopic______________________
original______________________
origination______________________
competition______________________
confidential______________________
toleration______________________
personnel______________________

Audio-Activity 7.3. Listening for Stress in Words and Word Sets (CD 2, Track 30)

Transcribe each word with appropriate reduced vowels, and mark primary stresses where they occur. There are six words. Check your answers carefully.

1. _______	2. _______
3. _______	4. _______
5. _______	6. _______

Answers

ˈpræktəkl̩	præktəˈkælɪt̬i
dʒiˈɑgrɪfi	dʒiəˈgræfɪk
ˈkɑrʔwil	pɚsəˈnɛl

Compound Words and Stress Placement

A common way of making new words in English is by compounding. Two old words are joined into a new word. So *green* and *house* are joined to form the compound word *greenhouse*. Generally, the first word receives the high pitch point, and, therefore, the primary stress, whereas the step-down in pitch occurs on the second element. Nevertheless, we cannot say that the second element is unstressed. It receives a secondary stress, a clear stress, but a little weaker than a primary stress. The IPA uses a lowered version of the primary stress symbol to represent this weaker strong stress: /ˌ/. *Greenhouse* consists of /ˈgrin/ plus /ˌha͜ʊs/, the first syllable getting the primary stress and the second syllable a weaker version of a strong stress. Although there is usually only one primary stress, there can be several secondary stresses in a compound word just as there can be multiple levels of non-primary (secondary) stress in a phrase or sentence. Once again, the pitch test shows these levels of stress, in that primary stress occurs on the pitch jump, with weaker stress on the steps down from this point.

Transcription Exercise 7.11. Compound Words

Transcribe these items using both kinds of stress marks.

showboat_______________	windowshop_______________
greenhouse_______________	Whitehouse_______________
drawbridge_______________	lawnmower_______________
toadstool_______________	flashlight_______________
lighthouse_______________	lifeboat_______________
spaceship_______________	wastebasket_______________
sharkskin_______________	tightrope_______________
billfold_______________	litterbug_______________

Audio-Activity 7.4. Listening for Stress in Compound Words (CD 2, Track 31)

Transcribe what you hear, paying careful attention to primary and secondary stress in these compound nouns and words. There are six items.

1. _______	2. _______
3. _______	4. _______
5. _______	6. _______

Answers

ˈwa͜ɪtˌha͜ʊs	ˈfa͜ɪnl̩ ɪgˌzæm
ˈʃoˌbot	ˈhæŋgrɪˌned
ˈgrosriˌstɔr	ˈkɑlɪdʒˌ studn̩t

Stress Placement With Modifier Plus Noun

When an adjective precedes a noun, it will usually receive secondary stress. To see how this works, compare *a green house* (/əˌ grin 'haʊs/) to the transcription of compound words such as *a greenhouse* as discussed in Transcription Exercise 7.11, that has its pitch jump (primary stress) on *green* (/'grinˌhaʊs/). (*Note*: When such words are spoken with two primary stresses, they are called *spondee words* and are used in the testing of hearing.) Only when a speaker wants to emphasize the importance of the modifier will it receive primary stress.

The Pitch Test Applied to the Three Kinds of Word Combinations

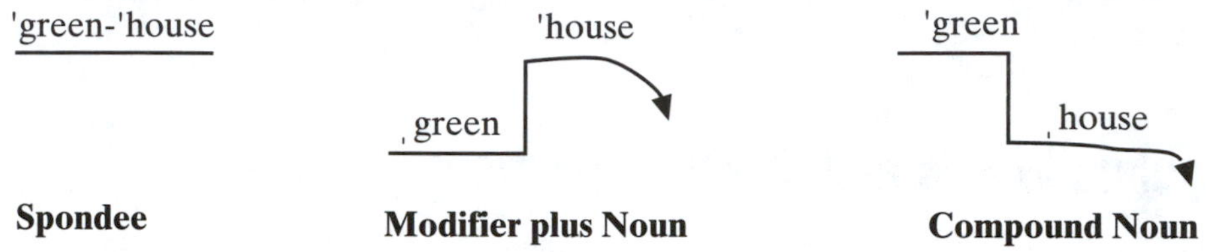

Transcription Exercise 7.12. Compound Words and Modifier Plus Noun Combination

Transcribe the following, remembering to place primary stress on the first noun in compound nouns and on the noun following the modifier in modifier plus noun combinations. As usual, use your own dialect as a basis for transcription.

a lighthouse________	a light lunch________
a short nap________	a shortstop________
the paper boat________	the paperback________
a slow train________	a slowpoke________
to play house________	a playhouse________
a longhorn________	a large horn________

Transcription Exercise 7.13. Special Emphasis on Modifier Plus Noun Combinations

In American English, subtle meanings may be added to speech by the use of special emphasis, the use of a pitch jump (primary stress) to add our own interpretation. In such cases, we may elect to place primary stress on the modifier rather than the noun. Transcribe the following modifier plus noun combinations as indicated, paying attention to the subtle shift in meaning with the change in primary stress.

Primary Stress on the Noun	Primary Stress on the Modifier
a poor outlook________	________
a leaky lifeboat________	________
a positive attitude________	________
a lousy day________	________

Audio-Activity 7.5. Listening to Modifier Plus Noun Combinations (CD 2, Track 32)

Transcribe what you hear very carefully, paying attention to the way that primary stress is used. There are five items to transcribe.

1. ________ 2. ________
3. ________ 4. ________
5. ________

Answers

əˌ grin'haʊs	ðə 'grinˌ haʊs
ə 'hɑrd ˌprɑbləm	ðəˌpepɚ 'bot
ðə 'pepɚˌbæk	

Transcription Exercises 7.14. Review

Transcribe these words. Remember to put into practice the points drilled in this and previous sections of this workbook.

obituary ________	aborigine ________
transcribe ________	blameworthy ________
unquenchable ________	Republican ________
embroider ________	agriculture ________
cold temperature ________	texture ________
wardenship ________	ordinary ________
inhibitor ________	management ________
fledgling ________	domesticate ________
melancholy ________	Dracula ________
liquefy ________	acquiescence ________
betrayal ________	cottontail ________
testimonial ________	bloodthirsty ________
statistical ________	pinnacle ________
smattering ________	smorgasbord ________
nonsense ________	sandpaper ________
independent ________	stethoscope ________
measuring tape ________	irregular ________
groceries ________	wintergreen ________
undergraduate ________	engorge ________
clergy ________	unconscious ________
populous ________	executioner ________
clinician ________	a large computer ________

Audio-Activity 7.6. Auditory Review of Transcription Principles (CD 2, Track 33)

This activity consists of some of the words in Transcription Exercise 7.14, reviewing some of the transcription principles you have been learning. There are six items.

1. ______	2. ______
3. ______	4. ______
5. ______	6. ______

Answers

ˈdrækjɪlə	ˈblʌdˌθɚsti
ˌɛksəˈkju̯ʃənɚ	ˈsænˌpepɚ
ˈmɛʒɚĩŋˌ tep	kləˈnɪʃən

SECTION 8

Transcribing More Allophonic Variations: Diacritics

Introduction

A diacritic is a mark used together with a phonetic symbol to modify the way the sound represented by that symbol is pronounced. You have already been using certain diacritics in your transcriptions. To show the intervocalic /t/ with partial voicing, you used /t̬/, and in a sense, the mark under the syllabics is a kind of diacritic. You have also been introduced to two other marks: the devoicing diacritic, used with /z̥/ for final-position devoicing, and the tilde /˜/ placed over vowels to show nasalization.

Phoneticians do not use diacritics to make their transcriptions look interesting or advanced. Rather, these extra markings are used sparingly and only when they are required to make a point or to adjust a phonetic symbol so that a particular feature of speech might not be lost. The student of phonetics, therefore, should not use diacritics as salt and pepper to season transcriptions, but only when nothing else will do.

You might question why phoneticians need diacritics. In cases where no standard phonetic symbol exists, diacritics are affixed to those symbols to add precision to the transcription. In the exercises in this section, only the most widely used diacritics are drilled, those that show the effects of assimilation or make a particular point about how American English may be spoken. First, a case from Section 3(3.4), in which syllabics are used in relation to homorganic stops, is expanded. Next, the nasal release of stop consonants and assimilated nasality of vowels is presented. The diacritics used to show stop release with or without aspiration, lip-rounding, lengthening, and dentalization are also examined.

Nasal Assimilation of Vowels and Stop Consonants

As demonstrated, a nasal consonant may affect the quality of the vowel that occurs with it in that some nasal resonance invades the surrounding sound. The term nasal assimilation is used to describe this phenomenon. Compare the pronunciation of the *a* in *man* and *bat*. The tilde, /˜/, would be the appropriate diacritic to use in the transcription of *man* over the /æ̃/ because it is nasalized, but not in *bat* for which the velopharyngeal mechanism remains closed, thus permitting little, if any, nasal resonance. There are pronunciations in American English in which a degree of nasal release on the stop consonants is typical, as in *rob 'em* and *stop 'em*. Such nasalization of the stops will occur when they are followed by a nasal syllabic, in which case the tilde is placed over the stop, for example, /stɑp̃m̩/.

Transcription Exercise 8.1. Transcribing Nasalized Sounds

Use the /˜/ over the nasalized vowel or the appropriate stop consonant that is produced with nasal airflow. Use syllabics wherever possible.

rob 'em__________	dip 'em__________
man__________	banter__________
tap 'em__________	written__________
splittin'__________	keep 'em__________
sudden__________	ridden__________
can__________	ointment__________
dance__________	mountain__________
maintenance__________	fountain__________

Audio-Activity 8.1. Listening for Nasalized Vowels (CD 2, Track 34)

Complete Transcription Exercise 8.1. Then use the diacritic for nasalization where appropriate on the vowels and stop consonants in the following six words and nonsense items.

		Answers	
1. ______	2. ______	ˈstap̃m̩	ˈsʌ̃mp̃m̩
3. ______	4. ______	ˈrɪtən	ˈrɪt̃n̩
5. ______	6. ______	ˈkæ̃n	ˌpæ̃ŋˈkæp̃m̩

Learning Activity: Acoustic Properties of the Voiceless Stops

An intensity-by-frequency or power spectrum for a sound provides an instantaneous picture of the loudness of a speech sound, shown vertically from low (at the bottom) to high (at the top). Its pitch, shown horizontally, ranges from low (on the left) to high (on the right). Although it is not practical to make an intensity-frequency display for the stopped portion (the closure) for the voiceless stops, the following release with aspiration does contain loudness and pitch information. Therefore, for each of the stop consonants there is a dome or area of greatest loudness (energy). First look in Chapter 5 of *Applied Phonetics (AP)* for the spectra for each of the voiceless stops (Division 8A), and read the Acoustic Description (8C), too. Then do the Learning Activity—it will help you to see the relationship between aspiration and the intensity-frequency (I/F) composition of the voiceless stops.

Learning Activity 8.1. Mapping Power (Intensity/Frequency) Spectra

On the empty I/F spectrum below, draw in an approximate line for *each* of the voiceless stops. You will notice that arrows appear at three points in the spectrum. Make sure that an area of acoustic energy appears at one of these arrows for each stop consonant. There will be a different area of energy prominence for each sound. Draw a dotted line for /k/, a connected line for /t/, and a dashed line for /p/. When you have done this, circle the correct word in the questions that follow.

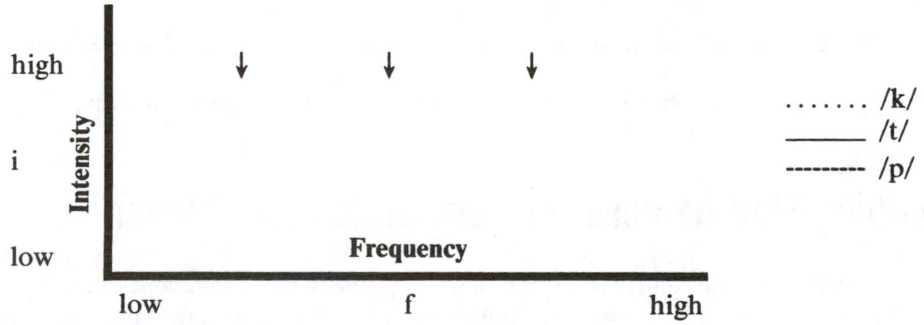

a. Where is the greatest intensity concentration for /p/?	Low	Mid	High
b. Where is the greatest intensity concentration for /t/?	Low	Mid	High
c. Where is the greatest intensity concentration for /k/?	Low	Mid	High

Note: In earlier attempts to determine the distinctive features for the sounds of English (Jakobson, Fant, & Halle, 1952), these areas of spectral energy were important. For those sounds with low prominence, the term +Grave was used; for high prominence, the term +Acute was assigned; and those sounds having centrally located energy were referred to as +Compact. How would the stops be differentiated under this system?

Learning Activity 8.2. The Stops and Voice Onset Time (VOT)

A stop consonant represents a momentary cessation of speech as the articulators come together and a pressure build-up occurs prior to release. If the time from the moment of closure to the release of the stop for a following vowel or voiced consonant is measured, the onset of voicing can be plotted and thus the voice onset time (VOT) can be derived (Klatt, 1975). Read the information in Chapter 5 of *AP* on VOT, found in the Introduction (pp) and in Division 8G, Voice Onset Time for each sound. Then complete the table and answer the questions that follow.

2.3a. Voice onset time for the initial position stops

Voiceless Stops	VOT (msec)	Voiced Stops	VOT (msec)
/p/	________	/b/	________
/t/	________	/d/	________
/k/	________	/g/	________

2.3b. Answer the following questions by circling T for true or F for false

T F 1. The voiceless stops have shorter VOTs than the voiced stops.

T F 2. The bilabial stops have shorter VOTs than the alveolar or velar stops.

2.3c. Voice onset time for the stops in initial position clusters

	s + Voiceless Stop + r		Voiced Stop + r	
Bilabial	/spr/	______	/br/	______
Alveolar	/str/	______	/dr/	______
Velar	/skr/	______	/gr/	______

2.3d. From the values that you found for the table in 2.3c, answer the following questions by circling T for true or F for false

T F 1. Clusters with s+voiceless stop+r have similar VOTs to voiced stop+r clusters.

T F 2. The bilabial stops have longer VOTs than either alveolar or velar stops.

■ Transcribing Stop Release With and Without Aspiration

The stop consonants are quite similar in terms of the allophonic patterns into which they fit. Review them in Chapter 5 in *Applied Phonetics* to see how similar they are. For example, the voiceless stops are almost always aspirated when they occur in word-initial or primary stressed positions. Phoneticians show aspiration in one of two ways: with a raised (superscripted) /^{h}/ or a /^{c}/, placed just after and slightly above the /p/, /t/, or /k/, for example, /p^{h}/ or /p^{c}/. We prefer the superscript /^{c}/ to show aspiration partly because it is congruent with the symbol for release without aspiration discussed below. The voiced stops /b/, /d/, and /g/ do not share this feature. In fact, when /p/, /t/, and /k/ are not aspirated where expected, as in the speech of non-native speakers, they are often perceived as their voiced cognates. In unstressed syllables, and especially in consonant blends (or clusters), the voiceless stops are released but not heavily aspirated. This is shown with the superscript backward c, /^{ɔ}/, also placed after and slightly above the symbol by most transcribers. Once again, this diacritic only applies to the voiceless stops. Finally, it is common for speakers of American English not to release the stops in word-final position. When another consonant follows, the stop may not be released as such, but blended into the next consonant. Transcribers show nonrelease or release into the next sound by the use of a superscript / ¯/ placed after and slightly above the stop. This feature applies to both voiceless and voiced stops.

Transcription Exercise 8.2. Transcribing Initial-Position Aspiration

Pay particular attention to the transcription of the stops in this exercise. Notice that the stops at the beginning of stressed syllables have longer VOTs than stops in other syllables.

page____________________ Kenneth____________________

peace____________________ tablecloth____________________

tacky____________________ kissed____________________

pamphlet____________________ tournament____________________

curve____________________ torture____________________

pause____________________ Cathy____________________

Audio-Activity 8.2. Listening for Aspiration of Initial Position Stops (CD 2, Track 35)

In this activity, show initial position aspiration in the six words that you hear.

1. _______ 2. _______
3. _______ 4. _______
5. _______ 6. _______

Answers

ˈp^{c}ɑrʃl̩	ˈt^{c}iˌkɛt̬l̩
ˈk^{c}ænsl̩	ˈt^{c}ot̬l̩
ˈk^{c}ænəˌlop	ˈp^{c}ʌfi

Transcription Exercise 8.3. Transcribing Initial-Position Aspiration

Transcribe the following, showing release of the stop, but without the heavy aspiration typical of initial-position production for the voiceless stops.

scab____________________ stooge____________________

straight____________________ misunderstood____________________

scattered____________________ asking____________________

spent____________________ whisper____________________

responsive____________________ astonish____________________

Audio-Activity 8.3. Listening for Release Without Heavy Aspiration (CD 2, Track 36)

In this activity, listen for and transcribe appropriately the release without heavy aspiration in these six words.

		Answers	
1. _______	2. _______	ˈstᵓʌmbl̩	dɪˈstᵓɝbd
3. _______	4. _______	ˈspᵓɔrtsˌkᵓæstᵓɚ	ˈspᵓitʃləs
5. _______	6. _______	ˈskᵓut̬ɚ	skᵓəˈmæt̬ɪk

Transcription Exercise 8.4. Transcribing Stops Without Release

Transcribe these words, showing nonrelease of the stop at the end of the word, or before another releasing consonant.

afloat______________________	namesake______________________
negate______________________	misplace______________________
sportscast______________________	supermarket______________________
bagpipe______________________	backstop______________________
marigold______________________	iceberg______________________
rock garden______________________	lip service______________________

Audio-Activity 8.4. Listening for Stops Without Release (CD 2, Track 37)

In this activity, show that the final stops in the following eight words are not released. Listen very carefully and pay attention to the way the preceding vowel is terminated. The last two words in this set demonstrate the nonrelease of the stop before another consonant. For items 9 through 12, use all of the diacritics for release/nonrelease of the stops as appropriate.

		Answers	
1. _______	2. _______	ˌsupɚˈsɑnɪk¯	ˈwa͜ɪz̥kræk¯
3. _______	4. _______	ˈlænz̥ˌkep¯	ˈbæt̬l̩ˌʃɪp¯
5. _______	6. _______	ˈla͜ɪfˌbot¯	ˈmunˌla͜ɪt¯
7. _______	8. _______	æk¯ˈtɪvət̬i	ˈkæp¯ˌsa͜ɪz̥
9. _______	10. _______	ˈstᵓɑp¯ˌsa͜ɪn	ˈkᶜʌstᵓəˌmɛri
11. _______	12. _______	ˈpᶜɛskᵓinəs	ˌɛk¯spᵓɛk¯tɚənt¯

Devoicing of Liquids After Voiceless Stops

The American English /r/ and /l/ become devoiced in blends with the initial position voiceless stops, /p, t, k/. The aspiration causes the liquid to become a fricative and the VOT is lengthened until the following vowel becomes voiced. With voiced stops, these sounds maintain their voicing feature. Also, /r/ and /l/ remain voiced following voiceless stops that are preceded by /s/ because the air needed for the friction is used previously by the /s/. Compare *print* and *sprint, platter* and *splatter*. Then, compare *train* and *drain, plaque* and *black*.

Transcription Exercise 8.5. Devoicing of Liquids

Transcribe, paying attention to the possible devoicing of /r̥/ and /l̥/ in these words. Check your transcriptions for the first three items in each column in Appendix B.

grain______________________	crane______________________
sprain______________________	tractor______________________
placemat______________________	bloodmobile______________________
precious______________________	approval______________________

crater______________	sprinkler______________
professional______________	stretcher______________

Audio-Activity 8.5. Listening for Devoiced Liquids (CD 2, Track 38)

Complete Transcription Exercise 8.5, then use the appropriate diacritic to show that the liquids are voiceless in the 10 words that you hear.

1. _______	2. _______	'pr̥ɛʃɚ	'tr̥ɑpɪk
3. _______	4. _______	kr̥ə'steʃən	'kl̥ʌbˌha͜ʊs
5. _______	6. _______	'pr̥a͜ɪvəsi	rɪ'tr̥iv
7. _______	8. _______	'pl̥ækɚd	ɪŋ'kr̥ɛdəbl̩
9. _______	10. _______	sɪm'pl̥ɪsət̬i	ɪŋ'kl̥udəbl̩

(Answers in the right-hand columns.)

Differentiating Clear l [l̦] as in *Leak*, Dark l [ɫ] as in *Lock*, and Velar l [ʟ] as in *Milk*

The /l/ sound is highly variable in American English and, therefore, treated differently by phoneticians. Here is an approach that may help you to understand this variability. Quite often /l/ may be produced in positions that differ from its usual alveolar placement (the clear l [l̦]) as heard in *leak* [l̦ik]. Compare this pronunciation to the retracted (palatalized) dark l [ɫ] in *lock* [ɫak], for which the tongue front contacts the hard palate behind the alveolar ridge. When it occurs, the dark l [ɫ] is the result of assimilating the /l/ to a following back vowel as in *law* [ɫɔ] or to a preceding back consonant, as in *glove* ['gɫʌv]. Now, pronounce the word *milk* and notice that if tongue contact occurs, it will be with the soft palate (or velum). This is the velar l as in *milk* ([mɪʟk]). This version of /l/ is frequently found as the releasing sound in consonant clusters (compare the /l/ sounds in *slick* [sl̦ɪk] and *silk* [sɪʟk]). The velar l may also follow vowels (including r-colored vowels) at the ends of words in American English, as in *curl* [kɝʟ] and *eel* [iʟ]. In such contexts, tongue contact with the velum is unnecessary. The syllabic l may be transcribed as [ɫ̩] or [ʟ̩].

Transcription Exercise 8.6. Transcribing Various /l/ Allophones

a. Transcribe these words using the clear l [l̦].

fleet______________	develop______________
slit______________	liability______________
lemon______________	leash______________
chili______________	ballet______________
collision______________	ledge______________

b. Transcribe these words using the dark l [ɫ].

glider______________	clipboard______________
parlor______________	column______________
follows______________	salute______________
mortal______________	huddle______________
global______________	catalog______________

c. Transcribe these words using the velar l [ʟ].

kelp____________________

bulky____________________

filthy____________________

polka____________________

spool____________________

twirls____________________

sculptor____________________

milkshake____________________

talcum____________________

already____________________

d. Transcribe these words using your own pronunciation as a guide. Use the allophones of /l/ as appropriate. Check your transcriptions to the first two items in each column in Appendix B.

linseed oil____________________

illegal____________________

labial____________________

Glendale____________________

calculator____________________

linoleum____________________

glide plane____________________

lonely wolf____________________

■ Assimilated Lip-Rounding

At times phoneticians want to show that the lips were rounded for the production of a usually unrounded sound. No one would describe /k/ as rounded, but in the word *creek*, there is definite lip-rounding, due to the influence of the rounded /r/. Lip-rounding, then, is the result of assimilating an unrounded sound to a rounded one, whether it is a consonant or a vowel. The diacritic is quite logical, a small /w/ under the newly rounded symbol: /k̼rik/.

Transcription Exercise 8.7. Rounding

In these words, use the diacritic for lip-rounding where possible. Do not mark sounds that are naturally rounded.

quack____________________

trachea____________________

graceful____________________

threatening____________________

serviceable____________________

globe trotter____________________

crackers____________________

fragrance____________________

although____________________

melodrama____________________

located____________________

snow drift____________________

Audio-Activity 8.6. Listening for Rounding (CD 2, Track 39)

After you have completed Transcription Exercise 8.7, transcribe the following eight words, marking sounds that are rounded because of the phonetic environment in which they occur.

1. ________
2. ________
3. ________
4. ________
5. ________
6. ________
7. ________
8. ________

Answers

ˈk̼wɒʃt	ˈsæŋˌg̼wɪn
ˈt̼resəbl̩	ˈĩŋˌk̼wɛst
ˌk̼ruˈsed̼ɚ	ˈha͜ɪd̼rəˌplen
ˈɛrk̼ræft	ˈd̼rɒˌb̼rɪdʒ

Lengthening of Abutting Sounds

The diacritic for lengthening is /ː/. In normal speech, when the same sound arrests one syllable and releases the next, lengthening usually results. Compare: *Stop them* to *Stop pushing*. The /p/, if lengthened, would be transcribed /pː/, not twice. A problem with using this diacritic is knowing where to place the stress marker. For this reason, sometimes it is better to double the consonant to show exactly where primary stress occurs. Compare: /ˈstɑpːʊʃɪŋ/ to /ˌstɑp ˈpʊʃɪŋ/.

Transcription Exercise 8.8. Lengthening

Transcribe these combinations showing lengthening where appropriate. For this exercise, do not worry about secondary stress marker placement. Use /ː/.

good days________________	leave Vinny________________
top production________________	some Monday________________
this Saturday________________	thank Karen________________
elect Tom________________	these zones________________
attack cat________________	hair-raising________________

Audio-Activity 8.7. Listening for the Lengthening of Sounds (CD 2, Track 40)

When you have completed Transcription Exercise 8.8 and understand the use of the diacritic for lengthening, listen to and transcribe the following six items.

1. _______	2. _______
3. _______	4. _______
5. _______	6. _______

Answers

ˈkrepːepɚ	dɪsˈmɪsːæm
ˈɝ̂nːa͜ɪn	ˈspɛlːɪkwəˌdet
ˈθæŋkːɛrɪn	ɪˈlitːæksˌpeɚ

Dentalization of Alveolars Before Interdentals

Dentalization, placing the tongue on the teeth rather than on the upper gum ridge, is shown by placing a small tooth, /◌̪/, under the symbol for the dentalized sound. Dentalization may occur as the result of assimilation as when an alveolar sound shifts forward under the influence of an interdental sound.

Transcription Exercise 8.9. Dentalization

Transcribe the following items showing dentalization where appropriate.

unthinking________________	hyacinth________________
width________________	hundredth________________
synthesis________________	parenthesis________________
eleventh________________	breadth________________

Audio-Activity 8.8. Listening for Dentalization (CD 2, Track 41)

Transcription Exercise 8.9 acquainted you with the diacritic for dentalization. Use the appropriate diacritic in these six words.

1. _______	2. _______
3. _______	4. _______
5. _______	6. _______

Answers

ˈbɛt̪si	ˈkloð̌d̪
ˈwɪd̪θ	ˈmʌn̪θ
ˈha͜ɪt̪θ	ən̪ˈθɪŋkəbl̩

This Audio-Activity is the last for Section 8. It also concludes CD 2.

PART II
ADVANCED TRANSCRIPTION

SECTION 9

Transcribing Connected Speech

To this point, you have been transcribing speech at the word or phrase level. Now, the focus will be on longer units of speech. Fortunately, most of the principles that apply to words and phrases also apply to transcribing connected speech. Note, for example, that the word *superintendent* may be said with five syllables, as many syllables as the sentence, *Sue really loves John.*

■ Principles for Transcribing Stress in Connected Speech

There have been many methods proposed for transcribing stress placement in stretches of language longer than a simple or complex word. Here three principles of linguistic structure are put forth that can be used as a guide for transcribing phrases and sentences.

Before stating the first principle, a brief discussion of phrases is necessary. A *phonological phrase* is a unit of connected speech that ends with a pause (or technically, a juncture). For example, it is easy to see that there is a single phrase in the sentence, "John turned green." In contrast, there are at least three phrases in, "Strictly speaking, articulatory phonetics is different from acoustic phonetics, but it is also different from phonology." The phrases are: "strictly speaking," "articulatory phonetics is different from acoustic phonetics," and "but it is also different from phonology." Often in writing, although not in all cases, commas mark the junctures that normally occur between phrases in speech.

The *first principle of linguistic structure* is that in each phonological phrase there will be one syllable that will receive primary stress (the high pitch point). All other syllables will receive lesser degrees of stress. Therefore, *strict*, *tic*, and *al* would be logical syllables for primary stress in, "*Strict*ly speaking, ar*tic*ulatory phonetics is different from acoustic phonetics, but it is *al*so different from phonology."

The *second principle* is that nearly always the word selected by a speaker to receive primary stress will be a semantically important word. For example, content words (nouns, verbs, adverbs, or adjectives), question words such as *who*, *what*, and *why* in information-asking questions, and usually the part of the sentence that contains new information may receive primary stress. This principle cannot be applied mechanically because stress depends on a speaker's particular interpretation of a sentence, and we cannot predict which precise word will receive the main stress in a phrase. A corollary to this principle is that function words (the noncontent words) are unlikely candidates for primary stress. Examples of function words are articles (e.g., *the*), conjunctions (e.g., *and*), pronouns (e.g., *me*), and auxiliary verbs (e.g., *is*). For the sentence: "He answered a few questions," put primary stress on various words to get a feel for what seem to be natural and unnatural possibilities. Decide on a word, then jump up in pitch on the important syllable. As you vary the stress placement, decide how the meaning of the sentence varies.

The *third principle* for transcribing stress is that once you have decided which content word receives primary stress, you should put a secondary stress marker on the other content words in the phrase, usually on the same syllable that would receive primary stress if that word were being pronounced in isolation. For a polysyllabic content word in a larger phrase, you can ignore the other syllables. For any function word, no matter how many syllables it has, you can leave it unmarked.

Examples:

ˌdʒɑn ˌtɚnd ˈgrin (normal statement with *green* as new information)
ˈdʒɑn ˌtɚnd ˌgrin (emphasis on *John*)
hi ˈænsɚd ə ˌfju əv a͡ʊr ˌkwɛstʃənz (emphasis on the verb)
hi ˌænsɚd ə ˌfju əv a͡ʊr ˈkwɛstʃənz (emphasis on the noun)

Although you will later be given an opportunity to transcribe simple and complex sentences, we will begin our transcription practice with phrases rather than sentences.

Applying the Principles

Read the following proverb that is transcribed in General American dialect.

ə ˈlezi, ˌʃip ˌθɪŋks ɪts ˈwʊl, hɛvi

Assume that this sentence has two phonological phrases: "A lazy sheep" and "thinks its wool heavy." There are, therefore, two primary stresses with secondary stresses on the third, fourth, and seventh words. Stress placement varies from speaker to speaker and is tied to those words that are considered semantically important. The most meaningful words are usually stressed. Remember that stress is primarily a pitch phenomenon with loudness, duration, and perhaps quality also playing important roles. In the items that follow, use the pitch test discussed in Part I, Section 2. In marking the three levels of stress (there are probably many more) show primary stress on the syllable(s) with the high pitch jump and use reduced vowels in unstressed syllables. Then mark secondary stresses on the remaining content words. To make your transcription easier to read, you may wish to keep word boundaries (the spaces between words) even though in some cases, you may find it better to combine smaller words that blend together in the actual stream of speech.

Assignment of Stress in Phrases

As has already been shown, the International Phonetic Association (IPA) system permits three levels of stress applicable to words, phrases, and sentences: primary stress /ˈ/, secondary stress /ˌ/, and no stress (unmarked). In longer units, grammatical words such as conjunctions, articles, prepositions, and modals are usually given reduced stress. The content words such as nouns, verbs, adverbs, and adjectives are excellent candidates for primary stress. The remaining syllables often receive secondary stress. The pitch test helps in deciding where to place the stress marks in the short phrases that follow. Transcribers rarely need to show secondary stress beyond the word or phrase level.

Transcription Exercise 9.1. Transcribing Short Phonological Phrases

Use your own dialect as reference and mark stresses appropriately.

about an hour ______________	over the hill ______________
the boy's watch ______________	her pencil ______________
the man on the street ______________	in case of accident ______________
up against it ______________	he can swim ______________
she has to study ______________	scared to death ______________
began to fall ______________	to get sick ______________
obliged to quit ______________	ought to be over ______________

Transcription Exercise 9.2. Vowel Reduction and /u/, /ʊ/, *and* /j͜u/

When the high back tense vowel /u/ occurs before another vowel, liquid, or glide, it may be reduced to a lax /ʊ/ instead of the expected schwa. Thus, as an emphasized word, *to* is pronounced /tu/, but when it occurs without stress before a consonant, it usually becomes /tə/. Before a vowel, however, it may become /tʊ/ as when *to end* becomes /tʊ ɛnd/. The /j͜u/ diphthong may be affected in the same way, as when *you* is pronounced as /j͜ə/ before a consonant and /j͜ʊ/ before a vowel, liquid, or glide. When unstressed /ʊ/ occurs before a glide or liquid, it may or may not reduce to schwa. Note that although words like *could* and *should* appear to have the liquid /l/ following /ʊ/, it is not pronounced so that /ʊ/ may reduce to /ə/ in connected speech. Transcribe the italicized words using vowel reduction where possible. Not every italicized word in the exercise can be reduced. The stressed syllables are underlined and should receive the primary stress in your transcription.

to <u>win</u> ________________	*You* <u>did</u> it ________________
Can *you* <u>sing</u>? ________________	<u>*Wood*</u> is good ________________
He <u>wants</u> *to* run ________________	He *would* <u>live</u> here ________________
It *could* ex<u>plode</u> ________________	It *<u>oo</u>zes* ________________
to <u>an</u>*swer* ________________	*to* <u>be</u> or not *to* be ________________

Transcription Exercise 9.3. Marking Phonological Phrases

In the following passage from Shakespeare's *Hamlet*, draw a vertical line between each phonological phrase. Use a slightly slower than average rate of speech so that you can catch all of the phrases. Next, <u>underline</u> the syllable that receives primary stress in each phonological phrase. Although there is some variation from speaker to speaker on the exact choice of phrases, the ones that you select should closely approximate those in Appendix B.

To be or not to be, that is the question. Whether 'tis nobler in the mind to suffer the slings and arrows of

outrageous fortune or by opposing end them.

Contrastive Stress

Several principles for the general placement of stress in phonological phrases have been given: the first element of a compound word may receive the stronger stress; in a modifier plus noun combination, the noun may receive the stronger stress; and a monosyllabic function word is unstressed. However, each of these principles may be overridden by a further application of the Second Principle for Transcribing Stress in Connected Speech, which states that nearly always the word selected by a speaker to receive primary stress will be a semantically important word (special emphasis).

Everyone has heard how a good actor, by varying the placement of the primary stress, can wring many meanings from sentences. "Everyone knows that Jill IS a good cook," might be said if someone had raised a question about Jill's cooking. Or, "Everyone knows that Jill is a GOOD cook," might mean that in the class of good cooks, Jill is one of the best.

An example of a structure where the normal principles of stress placement are overridden is a sentence in which two words or phrases are contrasted, as in the sentence, "I like blue skies in the morning better than gray skies." Normally, *skies* would receive greater stress than either *blue* or *gray*, but because the modifiers contrast, they become semantically more important and receive special emphasis.

Transcription Exercise 9.4. Contrastive Stress

Transcribe these sentences to show contrastive stress where appropriate.

Although Carl went to Denver to meet his family, Marsha stayed home. ________________

____

Mary wanted a blue dress to wear to the prom, but bought a green one. ______________________

____

He wanted a large piece of pie, but ended up with a small one. ______________________

____

Although we wanted to meet her at the concert, he showed up instead. ______________________

____

Audio-Activity 9.1. Listening for Phonological Phrases, Contrastive Stress, and Vowel Reduction (CD 3, Track 1)

Locate CD3 that accompanies this workbook. Then transcribe these 10 phrases as they are pronounced on Track 1, attending to the information presented in Transcription Exercises 9.1 through 9.4.

		Answers
1.	______________	ˌgʊd ˈmɔrnɪŋ
2.	______________	ˈwʌt̬ ə ˌla͜ɪf
3.	______________	ˈpɪktʃɚ ˌpɚʃɪkt
4.	______________	ˈɪkˈskj͜uz ˌmi
5.	______________	ˈwʌˌt:a͜ɪm ˌɪz ɪt
6.	______________	du ˌj͜u ɪn ˈdʒɔɪ ˌðɪs
7.	______________	ʃi ˈhæz̥ tə ˌstədi
8.	______________	ˌðe ˌwɑnt ˈhɪm wɪθ ˌhɚ
9.	______________	ˌðe ˌwɑnəm wɪθ ˈhɝ
10.	______________	ˌdu əˈwe wɪθ̬ ˌɪt

Transcription Exercise 9.5. Daffy Definitions

Transcribe the following definitions, intended to be humorous. Use special symbols and diacritics when appropriate.

Interdentals: The sounds that occur between visits to the dentist.

____

Phonology: The study of parties, games, and other fun-filled activities.

____

Dialect: What characterizes another person's speech but not yours.

____

Isogloss: A cold front situated between two dialects.

____

Fricatives: Speech sounds with slow leaks.

____

Transcription Exercise 9.6. A Limerick to Transcribe

Transcribe this short humorous poem. Notice that the primary stress is determined by the rhythm of the verse.

An expert in dialects with fame ______________________________

Found for some, "caught" and "cot" are the same. ______________________

Also "pen" becomes "pin" ______

And "Ben" becomes "bin," ______

but for all, the word "Mame" is said "maim." ______

Audio-Activity 9.2. Listening to a Limerick (CD 3, Track 2)

Listen to this limerick a few times. Then transcribe it before you listen to it again. Check your transcription with the one we have provided.

A Limerick

______

______

______

______

______

Answer

ə 'jʌŋ, fɑnɪˌtɪʃɪnː emd̚, rɑd/

ˌtræn'skra̯ɪbd ɪn əˌweðɛtwəz, ɑd/

wən 'θɪŋ i ˌwʊdːu/

ðɛt̚ ˌmed̚'titʃɚz̥, kwa̯ɪˀ ˌblu/

wəz̥ tə' sʌbstɪtut̚ ˌθeʈ ɪ fŋr ˌjɑd//

Transcription Exercise 9.7. Transcribing Proverbs

1. It is only the people with push who have pull.

______

2. Confessions may be good for the soul, but they are bad for the reputation.

______

3. A proverb is a short sentence based on long experience. (Cervantes)

______

4. Minds are like parachutes; they only function when open.

______

5. People who fall in love with themselves will have no rivals.

______

Audio-Activity 9.3. Listening to Some Proverbs (CD 3, Track 3)

When you have completed transcribing the proverbs in Transcription Exercise 9.7, transcribe the following four proverbs from dictation. Some are paraphrases of those in Exercise 9.7.

Proverbs

1. ______
2. ______
3. ______
4. ______

Answers

1. ðə ˈbɛstˌ weˌ a͜ʊt / ˌɪz ˈɒlwez̥ˌ θru
2. ˈpipl̩ ˌhu ˌhæv ˌpʊl / ˈɑlso ˌɑr ˌnon tu ˌhæv ˌpʊʃ
3. ˌla͜ɪk ə ˈpɛrɪʃut / ˈma͜ɪnz ˌonli ˌfəŋkʃɪn ˌwɛn ˌopɪn
4. ə ˈfækt ər ˌla͜ɪf ɪz ðæt / iˈvɛntʃəli ˌa͜ʊr ˌlək ˌwɪl ˌtʃendʒ

Transcription Exercise 9.8. A Passage to Translate

In this adapted story by Aesop (1947) of "The Fox and the Grapes," note that phonological phrases and primary stresses are kept to a minimum. Sentences are set off with a single slash. Diacritics are also used sparingly.

> ˌmɪstɚ ˌfɑks wəz ˈdʒʌst əba͜ʊt ˌfæmɪʃt/ hi wəz̥ ˈθɝsti ˌtu/ so hi ˈkrɛpt ɪntʊ ə ˌvɪnjɚd/ ðə ˌsənra͜ɪpənd ˌgreps wɚ ˈhæŋɪŋ ɑn ə ˌtrɛlɪs əbəv ðe ˌgra͜ʊnd/ ðe wɚ ˈtu ˌha͜ɪ fɚ ɪm tə ˌritʃ/ hi ˈræn ən ˌdʒəmpt fɚ ðə ˌnirɪst ˌbəntʃ əv ˌgreps/ bət̬ i ˈmɪst/ əˈgɛn æn əˌgɛn hi ˌtra͜ɪd/ ˌstɪl hi kʊd ˈnɑt ˌritʃ ðə ˌləʃɪs ˌpra͜ɪz̥/ ˈwɔrn aʊt wɪθ hɪz ˌɛfɚts hi ˌlɛft̪ ðə ˌvɪnjɚd/ ˈwɛl hi ˌmət̬ɚd a͜ɪ ˈnɛvɚ ˌrili ˌwɑnɪd ðoz ˌgreps ˌɛniwe/ a͜ɪm ˈʃɔr ðe ɚ ˌsa͜ʊɚ/ ðe ˈprɑbli hæv ˌwɚmz ɪn əm ˌtu/

Transcription Exercise 9.9. A Passage for Transcription

Following the devices used earlier, transcribe this standard reading passage from Darley, Aronson, and Brown (1975).

My Grandfather

You wish to know all about my grandfather. Well, he is nearly ninety-three years old; yet he still thinks as swiftly as ever. He dresses himself in an old black frock coat, usually several buttons missing. A long beard clings to his chin, giving those who observe him a pronounced feeling of the utmost respect.

Audio-Activity 9.4. Listening to a Story (CD 3, Track 4)

Here is a synopsis of a famous passage called "The Young Rat." The author is unknown. First, listen to the entire passage. Then, transcribe, sentence by sentence. Check your transcription with ours when finished.

The Story

Title: ____________________

____
____
____
____
____
____
____
____

Our transcription:

Title: ˈɑrθɚ/ fɔrˈɛvɚ əndəˌsa͜ɪdɪd

ˈɑrθɚˌ wəz ə ˌræt ˌhu ˌhæd ˈgret̚ ˌdɪfɪkəlti ˌmekin dəˌsɪʒɪnz̥/ ˌwɛn ˌɪt wəz̥ ˈta͜ɪm tə ˌgofɚ ə ˌwɐk/ ɔr
ɛn ˈgedʒ ɪn səm ˌəðɚ ˌfən æk̚ ˌtɪvɪt̬i/ ˌhi ˌkʊd ˈnɛvɚ də ˌsa͜ɪd ˌwət:ə ˌdu//ˈɑrθɚ ɛn ɪz̥ ˌfrɛnz ˌlɪvd ɪn ə
ˈvɛri ˌold̚ ˌbɑrn// ˌɪt ˌwəz əˈ dendʒɚəs ˌples// ˈwʌn ˌde ˈɔl ðə ˌræts də ˌsa͜ɪdɪd̥ tə ˌmuv tʊə ˌsefɚ
ples/ bət̬ ˈɑrθɚ ˌdɪd n̩t ˌno ˌwɛðɚ ˌhi ˌʃʊd ˈliv ɔr ˌste// hi rɪ ˈtɝnd̚ ˌtu ˌhɪz̥ ˌhol tə ˌθɪŋk// ˈðæʔ ˌna͜ɪt/ðə
ˈbɑrn ˌfɛl tə ðə ˌgra͜ʊnd wɪθ ə ˈla͜ʊd̚ ˌkræʃ// ɪn ðə ˈmɔrnin/ ˌɑrθɚ wəz̥ ˌfa͜ʊnd ˈsɔrt̬ əv ɪn æn ˌsɔrt̬ əv
ˈa͜ʊt̬ əv ˌhɪz̥ ˌhol// ˌhɪz̥ ˈfa͜ɪnl̩ dɪ ˌsɪʒɪn ˌhæd̚ ˌbɪn ˈmed̚ fɚ ˌhɪm/ ˌba͜ɪ ði ˈold ˌbɑrn//

SECTION 10

Transcribing More Dialect Differences

Transcription Exercise 10.1. Dialect Differences for the Stops

There are some interesting dialect differences related to the production of the stop consonants. Before continuing with this exercise, become familiar with these few differences by reviewing the related material in Chapter 5 (Division 6C) in *Applied Phonetics (AP)*. Then, transcribe the following, using the appropriate forms of the stop consonant for the dialect requested (do not be concerned about the other features of the dialect that may influence the vowel or other consonants—just the stops). Remember that any particular speaker of a dialect may or may not fit these general patterns. We are all quite individualistic in our use of the dialect of our geographical region and culture. In this exercise, attend to such general features as dentalization in New York City (NYC) and devoicing and final consonant blend reduction in African American English (AA) or African American Vernacular English (AAVE).

Transcribe these words so as to reflect stop consonant variation in each dialect.

a. New York City Speech (NYC)

dentist____________________	deed____________________
contact____________________	tentative____________________
different____________________	temptation____________________

b. African American Vernacular English (AAVE)

deed____________________	left____________________
test____________________	contact____________________
good rule____________________	stopped____________________

Audio-Activity 10.1. Listening for Dialect Differences (CD 3, Track 5)

Recall that in some dialects, the alveolar stops may be dentalized, final stops may not occur, or fricatives may be lengthened to substitute for the stops. Complete Transcription Exercise 10.1, then transcribe the following features of dialects in the words provided. Listen carefully for the way the stops are produced and try to transcribe those differences. There are six items.

1. _______	2. _______
3. _______	4. _______
5. _______	6. _______

Answers

'd̪ɛnt̪ɪst̪	'dɛnɪs:
'tu ˌtɛs:	'gʊ: ˌn t:a̯ɪ
't̪ɛst̪əmənt̪	'θri ˌvɛs:

Transcription Exercise 10.2. Southern American Dialect and /ɔr/

In Southern American dialect, when the letter *o* is followed by *r* or another consonant except *t* or *d*, the tendency is to use /ɔ/ so that *cork* would be pronounced /kɔk/. However, when the letters *or* are followed by *-e*, *-d*, or *-t*, *or* often becomes /o͜ə/. In this case, *core, board*, and *torte* become /ˈko͜ə/, /ˈbo͜əd/, and /ˈto͜ət/ (Wise, 1957).

Due to the variability usually found within each dialect, it is understandable that exceptions to these rules abound. Transcribe these items into Southern American dialect as described here.

shore ______________	shored ______________
orbit ______________	fort ______________
sport ______________	torque ______________
fork ______________	store ______________
score ______________	cord ______________
sword ______________	afford ______________

Audio-Activity 10.2. Listening for Southern American Dialect (CD 3, Track 6)

Complete Transcription Exercise 10.2. Then transcribe the following six words, some of which were taken from that exercise so you can hear how the words may be pronounced by some speakers of SA dialect.

		Answers	
1. _______	2. _______	ˈɔbɪt	ˈso͜əd
3. _______	4. _______	ˈspo͜ət	ˈfɔdʒ
5. _______	6. _______	ˈskɔtʃ	ˈʃo͜ə

Transcription Exercise 10.3. Eastern American and Southern American Dialect and /ɔ͜ɪ/

In NYC speech (or more specifically, Brooklynese) and in some parts of the deep South, it is possible to hear /ɚ/ or a diphthongized /ɜ͜ɪ/ in words where /ɔ͜ɪ/ is followed by a consonant, /ɚstə/ or /ɜ͜ɪstə/ as in *oyster*. A help in making this difficult sound-symbol correspondence for the diphthongized /ɚ/ is to produce /ɚ/, but with no lip-rounding and with the glide to the high-front space for /ɪ/. Transcribe these dialect differences using both /ɚ/, and /ɚ/. Practice pronouncing both forms, with and without lip-rounding.

	With /ɝ/	**With /ɜ͜ɪ/**
loin	______________	______________
point	______________	______________
toiling	______________	______________
poison	______________	______________

Audio-Activity 10.3. Listening for Eastern American and Southern American Dialect (CD 3, Track 7)

Complete Transcription Exercise 10.3. Then transcribe these six words as may be pronounced in GA, EA, and SA. The words *foist* and *loin* illustrate these pronunciations.

		Answers	
1. _______	2. _______	ˈfɔ͜ɪst	ˈfɝst
3. _______	4. _______	ˈfɜ͜ɪst	ˈlɔ͜ɪn
5. _______	6. _______	ˈlɜ͜ɪn	lɝn

Transcription Exercise 10.4. Southern American Dialect and /ɔ͜ɪ/ Before /l/

In the South, when /ɔ͜ɪ/ is followed by /l/, there may be a shift from the diphthong to either the vowel /ɔ/ or a lengthened /ɔː/. Remember that the diacritic /ː/ signifies lengthening. Here, lengthening may replace the articulation of final /l/, as in *oil* (e.g., /ɔl/ or /ɔː/). Transcribe in Southern American, using /ɔ/ and lengthened /ɔː/. Use /l/ in the words in the first column, but do not transcribe it in the second column because you will be using lengthening instead. Practice saying what you have transcribed.

	With /ɔ/ (with /l/)	**With /ɔː/ (without /l/)**
boil	______	______
recoil	______	______
toil	______	______
spoil	______	______

Audio-Activity 10.4. Listening for a Feature of Southern American Dialect (CD 3, Track 8)

When you finish Transcription Exercise 10.4, transcribe these six words as they are pronounced in General American and in either form of Southern American. The words *boil* and *foil* will be used.

1. ______ 2. ______
3. ______ 4. ______
5. ______ 6. ______

Answers

ˈbɔ͜ɪᵊl	ˈbɔl
ˈbɔː	ˈfɔ͜ɪᵊl
ˈfɔː	ˈfɔl

Audio-Activity 10.5. Listening to Two Dialect Samples (CD 3, Track 9)

Listen to these two slightly stereotypical pronunciations of NYC and SA dialects. Transcribe what you hear and then compare your results with ours.

1. ______________________________

2. ______________________________

Answers

1. ð̪ə ˈd̪ɛnt̪ɪst̪ ˌkɔd̪̚ t̪ə ˌse/ ð̪æt̪ ˈkɔfi ɪz ˌɔfl̩ fə ma͜ɪ ˈt̪iθ̪
2. ɑ ˈtʃendʒd ði ˌɔl/ ˌæftə ˈθʌt̬i ˌmɑlz̥

SECTION 11

Transcribing Non-Native Speech

Foreign accent, its analysis and transcription, is one of the most interesting and challenging areas of phonetic study. The varieties of foreign accent are about as varied as the numbers of speakers. However, within the set of American English speech sounds, a subset emerges that almost universally causes problems. For example, vowels are given a "spelling pronunciation" in that they are produced with a vowel sound that is a close spelling counterpart; lax vowels, including reduced vowels, tend to be tensed; the interdental fricatives are produced without sufficient airflow or retracted from usual place of articulation; and a lack of sufficient lip-rounding results in problems with /r/ and /w/, in particular. Let us examine the scenarios that result from each of these cases, remembering that any one non-native speaker of English will not necessarily reflect all of the pronunciations discussed here or sound like the resulting transcriptions. The illustrative sentences in each exercise are transcribed in Appendix B.

Transcription Exercise 11.1. Tensing of Lax Vowels

A speaker of a language such as Spanish may replace the lax vowels with their tense counterparts so that /ɪ/ becomes /i/ and /ʊ/ becomes /u/. The reduced vowels may be pronounced like their alphabet letter equivalents; for example, the *a* in *above* as /e/. Transcribe the words in Exercise 11.1 twice—once to show the General American dialect on target pronunciation, then again to demonstrate the tensing of lax vowels and, as a result, having no reduced vowels. The sentence is transcribed in Appendix B of this workbook so that you can check your transcription.

	Target Pronunciation	Tensing of Lax Vowels
hilltop	______________________	______________________
chipmunk	______________________	______________________
pamphlet	______________________	______________________
textbook	______________________	______________________

Sentence: Mister Fox was just about famished and thirsty, too.

Target: ____

Tensing of vowels: ____________________________________

Audio-Activity 11.1. Listening for the Tensing of Lax Vowels (CD 3, Track 10)

In this activity you will hear a word spoken with a lax vowel. Transcribe it. Then, substituting the vowel's tense counterpart, transcribe what will be another word. You will then hear the word that results from this lax-to-tense shift. For example, if you hear *live* transcribe it, and then transcribe *leave*. You will then hear the word *leave*. There are five basic items.

	Lax	Tense	Answers	
1.	________	________	'bɛst	'best
2.	________	________	'kʊd	'kud
3.	________	________	'bɪn	'bin
4.	________	________	'stʊd	'stud
5.	________	________	'dɛt	'det

Transcription Exercise 11.2. Airflow on the Interdental Fricatives, /θ/ and /ð/

When place of articulation is maintained but there is insufficient airflow, dentalized /t̪/ and /d̪/ result. Transcribe these words to demonstrate this feature of accented speech. The dentalized /t/ will substitute for /θ/ and the dentalized /d/ for /ð/.

	Target Pronunciation	Dentalization of Interdental Fricatives
weather	____________________	____________________
thirty-three	____________________	____________________
pathologist	____________________	____________________
therewith	____________________	____________________

Sentence: The thimbles that Thurman threw bothered father.

Target: ____

Dentalization: ____

Audio-Activity 11.2. Listening for Insufficient Airflow on the Interdental Fricatives (CD 3, Track 11)

Complete Transcription Exercise 11.2. Note how a /t/ and /d/, at times dentalized, may substitute for the interdental fricatives. Intelligibility may be affected when a real word occurs as the result of this substitution. You will now hear some words pronounced with interdental fricatives. Transcribe these words. Then, transcribe the word that results from changing the interdental fricatives to a voiced or voiceless dentalized /t/ or /d/. For example, if you hear *there* you will transcribe it as pronounced. Then you will show the substitution by transcribing *dare*, marking the /d/ for dentalization with the appropriate diacritic. You will then hear the word *dare*. Remember to transcribe two words for every initial word that you hear. There are six items.

	Interdental	Dentalized	Answers	
1.	________	________	'tuθ	't̪ut̪̚
2.	________	________	'fɑðɚ	'fɑd̪ɚ
3.	________	________	'θa͜ɪ	't̪a͜ɪ
4.	________	________	'mɪθ	'mɪt̪
5.	________	________	'ðɛn	'd̪ɛn
6.	________	________	'brið	'brid̪

Transcription Exercise 11.3. Wrong Place of Articulation on the Interdental Fricatives

When there is sufficient airflow but the tongue is retracted, the result is the substitution /s/ and /z/ for /θ/ and /ð/, respectively. Transcribe the same words and the sentence in Transcription Exercise 11.2 to demonstrate this change.

Target Pronunciation	Wrong Placement of Interdentals
weather ________	________
thirty-three ________	________
pathologist ________	________
therewith ________	________

Sentence: The thimbles that Thurman threw bothered father.

Target: ________________________________

Wrong placement: ________________________________

Audio-Activity 11.3. Listening for Wrong Placement of Interdentals (CD3, Track 12)

Complete Transcription Exercise 11.3 where you learned that /s/ and /z/ may substitute for the interdental fricatives. Continuing as before, you will hear a word pronounced with an interdental fricative. Transcribe this word. Then transcribe an alternate word with an appropriate /s/ or /z/ substitution for the interdental fricative. After you have transcribed this word, you will hear it on the tape. There are six words.

	Interdental	s/z Substitution	Answers	
1.	________	________	ˈθɪk	ˈsɪk
2.	________	________	ˈmɪθ	ˈmɪs
3.	________	________	ˈbeðz̥	ˈbez̥ː
4.	________	________	ˈði	ˈzi
5.	________	________	ˈpæθ	ˈpæs
6.	________	________	ˈsa͜ʊθ	ˈsa͜ʊs

Transcription Exercise 11.4. Lack of Lip-Rounding

Lip-rounding is important to American English, a fact that many non-native speakers may fail to notice. As a result of spreading the lips, the /r/ is replaced by an alveolar flap /ɾ/ or trill /ɹ/, or by /l/, the unrounded liquid. Either a /v/ or voiced bilabial fricative /β/ is used in place of /w/, and /s/ and /z/ substitute for /ʃ/ and /ʒ/, respectively. Follow the instructions as you transcribe these words and sentences.

a. Transcribe the words and sentence using [ɾ] for /r/ in all positions.

Target Pronunciation	Use of [ɾ] for /r/
rowboat ________	________
respect ________	________
arrived ________	________
pirate ________	________

Sentence: The crimson roses grew over farmer Ross's residence.

Target: ________________________________

Use of [ɾ]: ________________________________

b. For those who substitute the lateral /l/ for /r/, such as speakers of Japanese, the change is seen most clearly in word-initial position and in consonant clusters. In medial- and final-word position, the /l/ may be omitted. Transcribe the same words and sentence as in 11.4a., but in *over* and *Farmer* (in the sentence), show the /r/ omission rather than the /l/ substitution.

Target Pronunciation	**Use of /l/ for /r/**
rowboat______________	______________
respect______________	______________
arrived______________	______________
pirate______________	______________

Sentence: The crimson roses grew over Farmer Ross's residence.

Use of /l/ or omission: ______________________________

c. A sound similar to /v/ (actually [β]) is common among speakers of some Germanic languages as a non-rounded substitution for /w/. Transcribe these words and sentence demonstrating the use of /v/ for /w/.

Target Pronunciation	**Use of /v/ for /w/**
watched______________	______________
wicker______________	______________
wonderful______________	______________
sandwich______________	______________

Sentence: We witnessed wigwams everywhere.

Target: ______________________________

Use of /v/: ______________________________

d. Now transcribe these words and sentences showing the substitution of unrounded /s/ for the slightly rounded /ʃ/, a common pronunciation that may be found in speakers of Chinese, Vietnamese, and Thai.

Target Pronunciation	**Use of /s/ for /ʃ/**
shatter______________	______________
shiny dish______________	______________
workshop______________	______________
eyelash______________	______________

Sentence: Shepherds should cautiously establish pawnshops.

Target: ______________________________

Use of /s/: ______________________________

e. Likewise, show the unrounded /z/ for slightly rounded /ʒ/ in these words and sentence.

Target Pronunciation	**Use of /z/ for /ʒ/**
measure______________	______________
visual______________	______________
division______________	______________
leisurely______________	______________

Sentence: Asia's unusual treasures gave visual pleasure.

Target: ______________________________

Use of /z/: ______________________________

Note: Other potential problems not practiced here include omission of ends of words, simplification of consonant clusters, and trilling of /r/.

Audio-Activity 11.4. Listening for Lack of Lip-Rounding (CD 3, Track 13)

Complete Transcription Exercise 11.4 (a to e) to learn the importance of lip-rounding on certain English consonants. When these sounds are produced without rounding, other words may result, thus altering intelligibility. Continue as before by listening to and transcribing, these six words containing a rounded consonant. Then change this sound to its closest unrounded companion and transcribe the new word. Finally, listen for the word that you just transcribed.

	Rounded	Unrounded	Answers	
1.	________	________	ˈwɝs	ˈvɝs
2.	________	________	ˈʃem	ˈsem
3.	________	________	kəmˈpoʒɚ	kəmˈpozɚ
4.	________	________	ˈrɒŋ	ˈlɒŋ
5.	________	________	ˈʃɔr	ˈsɔr
6.	________	________	ˈwɛnt	ˈvɛnt

Audio-Activity 11.5. Listening to Accented English (CD 3, Track 14)

This activity has two parts. First, transcribe into General American dialect these three sentences from Aesop's fable, "The Fox and the Grapes":

Mister Fox was just about famished. He was thirsty, too. So he crept into a vineyard.

____

____

____

Answers

ˌmɪstɚ ˌfɑks wəz ˈdʒʌst əˌbaʊ̯t ˌfæmɪʃt/

hi wəz̥ ˈθɝsti ˌtu/

ˌso i ˈkrɛpt ˌɪntu ə ˌvɪnjɚd

Now you will hear five non-native speakers of American English say these sentences. Transcribe each, noting, the patterns that have been discussed in previous activities.

1. This is a native speaker of Russian.

____

____

____

Answers

ˌmistər ˈfɔks wəz̥ ˈdʒʌst eˌbaʊ̯t ˈfemiʃt/

ˌhi ˈwʌz̥ ˌsəsti ˌtu/

ˈso ˌhi ˈkrɛpt ɪnˌtu e ˈvaɪ̯nɛjɑrt

2. This is a native speaker of Spanish.

Answers

ˌmist̪əɾ ˈfɑks wəz̥ ˌdʒəs ɛˌba͜ʊ ˌfɑmiʃ/

ˌhi ˈwʌz̥ ˌt̪ɚst̪i ˌt̪u/

ˌso ˌhi ˈkɾɛp ɪnˌt̪u ˌe ˈba͜ɪnjɑɾ

3. This is a native speaker of Japanese.

Answers

ˈmɪstə ˈhɑks wəz̥ ˈdʒʌst əˌba͜ʊt ˈfɑmiʃt/

ˌhi ˌwəz̥ ˈsʌsti ˈtu/

ˈso ˌhi ˈkrɛp ˌɪntu ˌɛ ˈba͜ɪjɑrd

4. This is a native speaker of Chinese.

Answers

ˈmɪsː ˌfɑks wəz̥ ˈdʒʌs əˌba͜ʊt ˈfemiʃɪd/

ˈhi ˌwəz̥ ˌθɛrsti ˈtu/

ˌso ˌhi ˈkrɛp ˌɪntu ˈwa͜ɪnjɑrt

5. This is a native speaker of Vietnamese.

Answers

ˈmɪstə ˈfɔks wəż̥ ˈdʒʌˀ əˌba͜ʊˀ ˈfɑmlɪst/

ˈhi ˈwʌz̥ ˌtəst̪i ˈtu/

ˈso ˈhi ˌhrɛpt ˌɪntu ə ˈva͜ɪnɛˈjɑr

SECTION 12

Transcribing Phonologically Disordered Speech

Attempts to devise a phonetic alphabet to use in transcribing disordered speech have not met with a great deal of success (but see Duckworth, Allen, Hardcastle, & Ball, 1990). In fact, the existing alphabet as presented in this text, with slight modification, has proved useful for transcribing such speech. For substitutions and omissions of speech sounds, the International Phonetics Association (IPA) alphabet does well. More diacritics or even adapted symbols might be needed for distortions of and additions to speech sounds. For transcribing phonologically disordered speech, as illustrated in the following exercises, the existing alphabet works satisfactorily.

In the space of this text, all the varieties of disordered speech cannot be covered, so, as for non-native speech, several broad examples are provided. For more information on speech-sound deviations, see Chapter 4 in *Applied Phonetics (AP)*. Most of the examples given here are common in utterances of toddlers under 2 years of age or in the speech of older individuals with intelligibility problems. The nontarget sentences are transcribed for you in Appendix B of this workbook.

■ Phonological Patterns Characteristic of Child Speech

Transcription Exercise 12.1. Cluster Reduction

When two or more consonants occur in a sequence, one or more will be omitted. Typically, liquids and fricatives are deleted, with a stop, nasal, or glide retained. Transcribe each item twice, once to show the target (or adult) pronunciation, then again to demonstrate the child pronunciation with cluster reduction.

	Target Pronunciation	Cluster Reduction
slipper	________________	________________
sneak	________________	________________
pretty	________________	________________
bleed	________________	________________

Please bring a clean spoon for the snack. (Transcribe the two versions of this sentence below.)

Target: ______________________________________

Cluster reduction: ______________________________________

Audio-Activity 12.1. Listening for Cluster Reduction (CD 3, Track 15)

This activity demonstrates that intelligibility may be affected when clusters are reduced and different words result. After reviewing Transcription Exercise 12.1 and when you are ready to begin, you will hear eight words with clusters. Transcribe these words; then transcribe a different word that may result from the reduction of the cluster. You will then hear the word that you transcribed. Answers are provided in case you need them.

Cluster	Reduction	Answers	
1. ________	________	ˈspaɪ̯	ˈpaɪ̯
2. ________	________	ˈblaɪ̯t	ˈbaɪ̯t
3. ________	________	ˈbrek	ˈbek
4. ________	________	ˈstɑr	ˈtɑr
5. ________	________	ˈklɪŋ	ˈkɪŋ
6. ________	________	ˈskop	ˈkop
7. ________	________	ˈplʌmp	ˈpʌmp
8. ________	________	ˈsnæk	ˈnæk

Transcription Exercise 12.2. Stopping

Stops are often substituted for continuants (nonstops). Typically the substituted stop has the same voicing characteristic and the same or similar place of articulation. In the transcription of these items, retain the same voicing and the same or nearest place of articulation for the substitute stop for each of the consonantal continuants.

Target Pronunciation	Stopping
vet________________________	________________________
fake________________________	________________________
zip________________________	________________________
sack________________________	________________________

Susie and Van saw four sheep at the zoo.

Target: ____

Stopping: ____

Audio-Activity 12.2. Listening for Stopping (CD3, Track 16)

In this activity you will hear eight words containing one or more nonstop consonants in initial or final position. Transcribe the word as pronounced. Then select a stop with the same voicing and general place of articulation as the nonstop consonant or consonants in the previous word and transcribe the new word. Next, you will hear the word that you transcribed. Note that some of these words will result in the same word when stopping occurs. For example, *mat, vat, math*, and *mass* may all be pronounced as *bat*. Repeat this activity until you understand each change that occurs.

Nonstop Sound	Stop Replacement	Answers	
1. ________	________	ˈfæt	ˈpæt
2. ________	________	ˈθɪk	ˈtɪk
3. ________	________	ˈves	ˈbet
4. ________	________	ˈmæn	ˈbæd

5. ________	________	'sɪk	'tɪk
6. ________	________	'zu	'du
7. ________	________	'sæt	'pæt
8. ________	________	'væn	'bæd

Transcription Exercise 12.3. Prevocalic Voicing

Some children produce only voiced consonants preceding vowels. Transcribe these items in a way that demonstrates prevocalic voicing. Use the diacritic for voicing, /̬/, under the appropriate stop consonant.

Target Pronunciation	Prevocalic Voicing
comb________________	________________
tea________________	________________
paint________________	________________
pecan________________	________________

Timmy took cookies to the party.

Target: ________________________________

Prevocalic voicing: ________________________________

Audio-Activity 12.3. Listening for Prevocalic Voicing (CD 3, Track 17)

Once you understand the concepts in Transcription Exercise 12.3, listen and transcribe the following six words. First, a word will be given containing one or more voiceless consonants. Transcribe what you hear. Next, change the voiceless sounds to their voiced counterparts and transcribe the new form. You will then hear what you just transcribed. Repeat this activity until all the changes are clear to you.

Voiceless Sound	Voiced Replacement	Answers	
1. ________	________	'taɪ̯m	'daɪ̯m
2. ________	________	'pɛr	'bɛr
3. ________	________	'pɑpi	'bɑbi
4. ________	________	'kækl̩	'gægl̩
5. ________	________	'fju̯	'vju̯
6. ________	________	'tɪkɪt	'dɪgɪt

Transcription Exercise 12.4. Assimilation

Children often substitute consonants that are similar in manner or place of articulation to another consonant in the word. One of the most common types of assimilation is labial assimilation, which involves substituting a labial consonant for a nonlabial consonant in a word that already has a labial consonant in it. In your transcription, retain the same manner and voicing that the target phoneme had for the substituted sound.

Target Pronunciation	Assimilation
dime ________________	________________
comet ________________	________________
tabby ________________	________________
smell ________________	________________

Tommy smiled as he put the cup on the table.

Target: ______________________________

Assimilation: ______________________________

Audio-Activity 12.4. Listening for Assimilation (CD3, Track 18)

Read about how nonlabial consonants may assimilate to labial consonants in words containing a labial consonant in Transcription Exercise 12.4. In this activity, only this kind of assimilation is studied, although you may read about other kinds in *AP*. As before, transcribe the word you hear; make the change, and transcribe the new form; then wait to confirm what you transcribed. There are six items.

Nonlabial Sound	Labial Replacement	Answers	
1. ________	________	'kɑp	'pɑp
2. ________	________	'tʌb	'pʌb
3. ________	________	'sem	'fem
4. ________	________	'bit	'bip
5. ________	________	'kʌp	'pʌp
6. ________	________	'kepɚ	'pepɚ

Transcription Exercise 12.5. Gliding

Children commonly substitute /w/ for other consonants, especially the liquids, /l/ and /r/. Some children substitute /j/, but this is less common than the /w/ substitution. Transcribe these items showing the substitution of /w/ for the liquids.

	Target Pronunciation	Gliding
laughed	______________________	______________________
rice	______________________	______________________
buffalo	______________________	______________________
arrest	______________________	______________________

Larry ran around the long lake.

Target: ______________________________

Gliding: ______________________________

Audio-Activity 12.5. Listening for Gliding (CD 3, Track 19)

Recall that gliding is the result of substituting, the /w/ or /j/ glides for the liquids, /r/ and /l/. Intelligibility may be impaired when a different word is produced by gliding. As before, transcribe the word you hear. Then transcribe the word that results by substituting a glide. You will then hear a confirmation of your second transcription. In this activity, use the /w/ glide as a substitute form for the first four and the yod as a substitute for the last four items. There are eight items in all.

Liquid	Glide Replacement	Answers	
1. ________	________	'ræg	'wæg
2. ________	________	ə'rek	ə'wek
3. ________	________	'let̬ɚ	'wet̬ɚ
4. ________	________	'rɛd	'wɛd

5.	________	________	ˈlɛt	ˈjɛt
6.	________	________	ˈlɑrd	ˈjɑrd
7.	________	________	ˈlɛs	ˈjɛs
8.	________	________	ˈlist	ˈjist

Audio-Activity 12.6. Listening to Samples of Childhood Phonological Patterning (CD 3, Track 20)

Here are some samples of childhood phonological deviations. Transcribe what you hear, keeping in mind the principles and features that you have learned.

1. This child uses gliding for the liquids.

   ____

2. This child reduces clusters.

   ____

3. This child uses several of the features described in this section.

   ____

Answers

1. ˈsizən ˌmin ˌwa͜ɪk ˈɒt̬ɪm æn ˈwɪntʊ æn ˈspwɪŋ æn ˈsʌmʊ
2. ˈpɪn ˀə ˌtɑp ˌte ˈĩə ˌbot
3. ə ˈkᶜ ʊˀ i ˌmɑ̃ˀə ˈlæˀ æˀˈɒd̪ʊ

■ Patterns That May Persist into Adult Speech

Transcription Exercise 12.6. The Frontal Lisp

For the frontal lisp, the articulation for /s/ and /z/ is shifted slightly forward (fronted), which causes these sounds to be dentalized while maintaining the stridency characteristic of /s/ and /z/. Although other symbols have been suggested, for this exercise simplify the task slightly by transcribing the frontal lisp with the diacritic for dentalization, [̪], placed under the standard symbol for /s/ or /z/.

	Target Pronunciation	**Frontal Lisp**
submerse	________________	________________
precipice	________________	________________
zebras	________________	________________
magazine	________________	________________

Sam's sister sells zinnias in summer.

Target: ____

Assimilation: ____

Transcription Exercise 12.7. The Lateral Lisp

To produce the lateral lisp, the tongue may be held in the general articulatory position for the clear /l/, but with sufficient lateral airflow to produce an audible fricative noise. One way to show this presence of stridency is to transcribe the lateral lisp for /s/ as [ls], marking the /l/ for devoicing—[̥]. For /z/, the lateral lisp is transcribed [lz]. The slur, [‿], is used to tie the digraph together.

	Target Pronunciation	Lateral Lisp
submerse	____________	____________
precipice	____________	____________
zebras	____________	____________
magazine	____________	____________

Sam's sister sells zinnias in summer.

Target: ____________________

Lateral lisp: ____________________

Transcription Exercise 12.8. Overuse of the Velar-l

You have already seen that the velar-l, [L], is quite frequent in American English. In Transcription Exercise 8.6 you learned that velar-l occurs as the beginning sound in /l/-clusters (*milk*) and when /l/ follows vowels (including r-colored vowels) at the ends of words (*curl* and *eel*). Some speakers generalize this pronunciation to phonetic contexts requiring either the clear l or the dark l (*leak* and *globe*) to produce [ʟik] and [gʟob]. When velar-l occurs in clusters with voiceless sounds, it will be transcribed with the diacritic for devoicing, [̥], underneath it as when *play* is pronounced [pʟ̥e].

	Target Pronunciation	Velar l
light	____________	____________
jello	____________	____________
literature	____________	____________
lamplighter	____________	____________
flippity-flop	____________	____________

Floyd let Lyle list the syllables

Target: ____________________

Velar l: ____________________

SECTION 13

Using Alternative Transcription Systems

Although dictionaries are very useful books, not very many of their editors use the International Phonetics Association (IPA) alphabet. Rather they use alternative transcription systems, some being more complex than others. Knowing the IPA version, however, will make translating between and among these phonetic alphabets somewhat easier as you will learn in the activities that follow. Before you begin, turn to Appendix C and review the alphabets as they compare to the one you now know. Then, complete the Learning Activity and Transcription Exercises that follow.

Learning Activity: Dictionary Alphabets

Learning Activity 13.1. Alternative Phonetic Alphabets

Answer the following questions based on Appendix C.

1. List the IPA symbols for the consonants that are also the same in all the dictionaries:

   ____

2. List the consonant symbols that are the same in all dictionaries, but different in the IPA:

   ____

3. Which dictionary uses vowel symbols that have the greatest difference from the symbols used in all the other dictionaries? ______________________
4. Which vowel symbol represents different vowels in different dictionaries?

   ____

5. Which dictionary allows the use of the same vowel symbol to represent two sounds that are treated distinctly in the IPA alphabet? ______________________

Learning Activity 13.2. Dictionaries and Stress Marking

The way stress is symbolized varies from one dictionary to another. Most, but not all, dictionaries show syllable divisions in words: some by putting hyphens at the end of a syllable; others by leaving a space at syllable ends. Several dictionaries use the IPA primary (ˈ) and secondary (ˌ) marks preceding the stressed syllables, for example, ˈin-venˌtor-y. Some dictionaries using the IPA symbols mark only primary stress, not secondary stress. Other dictionaries place a heavy acute accent (´) *after* the syllable with primary stress and a lighter acute accent (ˊ) after the syllable with second stress, for example, either in in´ven-tor-y or in´ven-tor´y. Another dictionary boldfaces the syllable with primary stress without marking secondary stress, for example, **in**-ven-tor-y.

For this exercise, notice the way different dictionaries show stress placement of the example words. Then mark the other words given in the same way in each column. In the last column, give the name of your dictionary and show the way its marks stress.

Word	American Heritage	Oxford American	Webster's Collegiate (10th)	My Dictionary
				________
confer	con-fer´	con-**fer**	con'fer	________
conference	con´fer-ence	**con-**fer-ence	'con-fer-ence	________
inventory	in´ven-tor´y	**in**-ven-tor-y	'in-ven,tor-y	________
blackbird	black´bird´	**black**-bird	'black,bird	________
system	________	________	________	________
delight	________	________	________	________
telegraph	________	________	________	________
baseball	________	________	________	________

Transcribing in Alternative Systems

Transcription Exercise 13.1. Alternative Phonetic Alphabets

The following words are transcribed as they would appear in various dictionaries. First, spell the word in standard English; then transcribe the word into your dialect, using the symbols of the IPA; and finally, tell which dictionary each transcription represents.

	Normal Spelling	IPA Transcription	Dictionary
1. buush- ĕl	________	________	________
2. fûr-thər	________	________	________
3. brə*th*-ər	________	________	________
4. but-ŏn	________	________	________
5. katl	________	________	________
6. kŏt	________	________	________
7. ăpl	________	________	________
8. skʉr-vē	________	________	________

Transcription Exercise 13.2. Key Words

Here are the key words for some of the consonant sounds listed in various dictionaries. Transcribe the words in the IPA. Then transcribe them in the system of your personal desk dictionary if it is one of the six listed in Appendix C. If it is not one of those listed, then pick the system of one of the dictionaries and transcribe each word.

Dictionary Used: ____

Word	IPA Transcription	Dictionary Transcription
1. paper	____________	____________
2. ticket	____________	____________
3. imbibe	____________	____________
4. dread	____________	____________
5. gag	____________	____________
6. fluff	____________	____________
7. thin	____________	____________
8. use (verb)	____________	____________
9. judge	____________	____________
10. sink	____________	____________

Transcription Exercise 13.3. Alternative Transcriptions

Transcribe each of the following words in the style of the dictionaries listed in Appendix C.

Word	AH	OA	WNW	W10C
1. freely	________	________	________	________
2. miss	________	________	________	________
3. thirst	________	________	________	________
4. tongue	________	________	________	________

Audio-Activity 13.1. Words to Compare (CD 3, Track 21)

To complete this activity, you will need to transcribe the following 10 words using the standard symbols of the IPA alphabet. Later, consult your dictionary to see how each word is transcribed there. Note the differences.

1 ________	2. ________
3. ________	4. ________
5. ________	6. ________
7. ________	8. ________
9. ________	10. ________

Answers

'renˌstɔrm	kəŋ'grɛʃənl̩
frɪ'nɛt̬ɪk	'ʃɑrpˌʃut̬ɝ
'tɝpənˌtan	ɪn'dʌldʒ
'vɛtr̥ɪn	ˌdɪspə'zɪʃɪn
ənɪm'pɔrˀn̩t	'ska͜ʊndrl̩

This is the last of the Audio-Activities and the end of CD3.

SECTION 14

Putting It All Together: A Review of General Concepts

Now that you have become proficient in phonetic transcription and can proudly wear the hat of a phonetician, it is time recap some of the knowledge and skills that you have learned. You should be very familiar with

- special terms that relate to phonetics.
- the classical descriptions of the major phonemes of American English.
- the special names given to specialized phonetic symbols.
- the major allophones of American English and their specialized names.
- the segmental notations (diacritics) and suprasegmental notations (prosodic).
- how to use *Applied Phonetics: The Sounds of American English* to answer phonetic questions.
- how to transcribe in broad (phonemic) and narrow (allophonic) versions.

Review Exercise 14.1. Special Terms Relating to Phonetics

Complete this vocabulary puzzle with the words matching each definition.

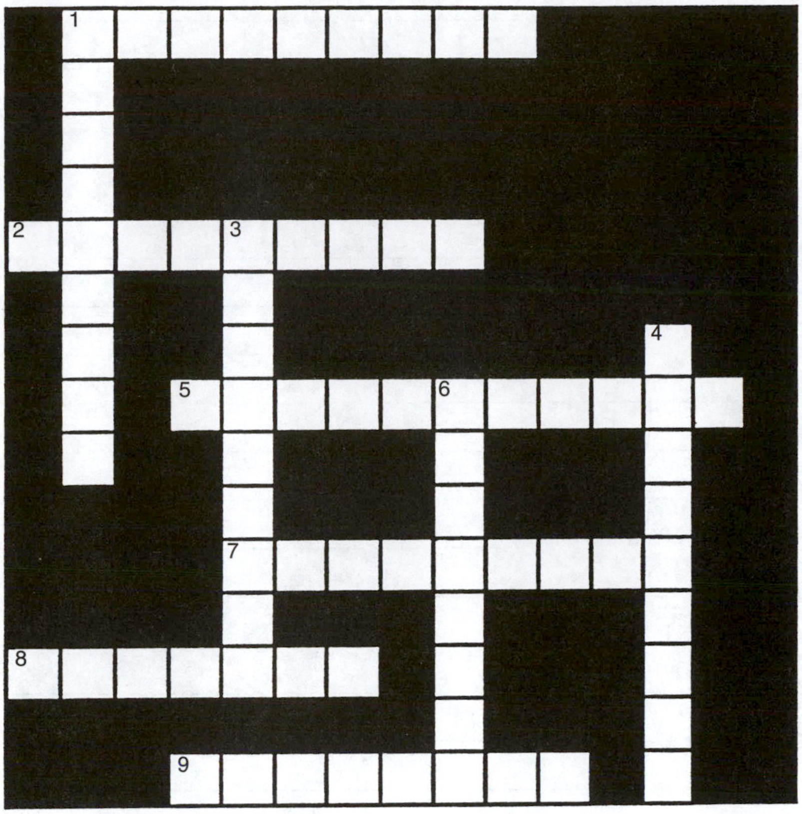

Across

1. Two vowels produced as one syllable
2. A sound produced with partial blockage of the breath stream
5. The writing and spelling system of a language
7. A variation of a phoneme
8. A variety of a language
9. The smallest linguistic unit of meaning

Down

1. A special mark used to change a sound feature
3. A stop-fricative combination
4. The study of speech sounds
6. A letter of the alphabet

Review Exercise 14.2. Classical Phonetic Descriptions

You are provided the Voice-Place-Manner descriptions for the American English phonemes for the consonants, and the physiological vowel diagram position for the distinctive vowels and diphthongs. For the vowel + /r/ combinations, a key word is provided. You should transcribe the appropriate symbol(s) in the space provided. You will want to review your flash cards before completing this exercise.

1. Voiceless Glottal Fricative: ______________________
2. Mid Front Tense Vowel: ______________________
3. Voiced Alveopalatal Liquid: ______________________
4. Voiceless Alveopalatal Affricate: ______________________
5. Voiceless Alveolar Stop: ______________________
6. High Front Lax Vowel: ______________________

7. Voiced Labiodental Fricative: ______________________________
8. Voiced Alveolar Nasal: ______________________________
9. Voiced Interdental Fricative: ______________________________
10. Mid Front Lax Vowel: ______________________________
11. Voiced Velar Stop: ______________________________
12. Voiced Palatal Fricative: ______________________________
13. Low Front Lax Vowel: ______________________________
14. Voiced Alveolar Stop: ______________________________
15. Voiced Palatal Glide: ______________________________
16. Voiced Alveolar Fricative: ______________________________
17. Voiced Alveolar Lateral: ______________________________
18. Lower Mid-Central-to-Back-Lax Neutral Vowel: ______________________________
19. Voiceless Bilabial Stop: ______________________________
20. Mid-Central /r/-colored Lax Vowel: ______________________________
21. High Front Tense Vowel: ______________________________
22. High Back Tense Rounded Vowel: ______________________________
23. Voiced Bilabial Stop: ______________________________
24. Mid Back Tense Rounded Vowel: ______________________________
25. Voiceless Alveolar Fricative: ______________________________
26. Voiceless Palatal Fricative: ______________________________
27. Low Back Lax Vowel: ______________________________
28. Voiced Alveopalatal Affricate: ______________________________
29. Rising Low Front to High Front Diphthong: ______________________________
30. Rising Low Front to High Back Diphthong: ______________________________
31. Voiceless Interdental Fricative: ______________________________
32. Rising Mid Back to High Front Diphthong: ______________________________
33. Voiced Bilabial Glide: ______________________________
34. Voiced Bilabial Nasal: ______________________________
35. High Front to High Back Diphthong: ______________________________
36. Voiceless Labiodental Fricative: ______________________________
37. Mid-Central Lax (Unstressed) Vowel: ______________________________
38. Voiceless Velar Stop: ______________________________
39. Mid-Central /r/-colored Tense Vowel: ______________________________
40. Voiced Velar Nasal: ______________________________
41. High Back Lax Rounded Vowel: ______________________________
42. Low Mid-Back Lax Rounded Vowel: ______________________________

The Non-phonemic Vowel + /r/ combinations

43. As in *car*: ______________________

44. As in *fear*: ______________________

45. As in *fair*: ______________________

46. As in *tour*: ______________________

47. As in *more*: ______________________

Review Exercise 14.3. Special Terms Used to Name Sounds

Again, review your flash cards, then provide the phonetic symbol for each name.

1. Theta: ______________________
2. Esh: ______________________
3. Eth: ______________________
4. Ash: ______________________
5. Ezh: ______________________
6. Eng: ______________________
7. Schwa: ______________________
8. Open-o: ______________________
9. Capped-a: ______________________ (as used with some of the diphthongs)
10. Jod: ______________________
11. Capped-i: ______________________
12. Flying-u: ______________________
13. Epsilon: ______________________
14. Stressed Schwa-r: ____________/Unstressed Schwa-r: ____________
15. Caret: ______________________

Review Exercise 14.4. Terms Used for Allophones

There are a few terms that we use to refer to specialized allophones. Transcribe them, based on their particular names as used in this workbook. Do not forget that some of these will require diacritics.

1. Glottal stop: ______________________
2. Intervocalic-t: ______________________
3. Alveolar tap (or flap): ______________________
4. Devoiced-z: ______________________
5. Reversed script-a: ______________________
6. Syllabic-m -n -ŋ -l: ______________________

Review Exercise 14.5. The Specialized Symbols: Diacritical (Segmental) and Prosodic (Suprasegmental)

Provide the specialized symbol used to show these phonetic adjustments made to standard phonemes in transcribing American English.

1. Lip rounding: ______
2. Aspiration: ______
3. Nonrelease: ______
4. Release without aspiration: ______
5. Dentalization: ______
6. Devoicing: ______
7. Nasalization: ______
8. Voicing: ______
9. Lengthening: ______
10. Slur: ______

Now provide the symbol used to show these prosodic changes.

1. Primary stress: ______
2. Secondary stress: ______
3. Short pause: ______
4. Long pause: ______
5. Falling pitch: ______
6. Pitch jump: ______

Review Exercise 14.6. Using the Appendixes in AP *to Answer Questions*

You have an important resource in *AP* to use in answering questions that require phonetic data. Here are some questions that you can answer in this way.

A. Using Appendix A in *AP* (p. 339), with help from Appendixes B and F (p. 341 and p. 360), answer the following questions.

1. What alphabet letter representing a stop is the most frequent of the consonant graphemes in English? ______
2. What alphabet letter representing the semivowels /w/, /l/, and /r/ is the most frequent in *written* English? ______
3. Rank order, from most to least frequent, the alphabet letters for the stop consonants (do not include either *c* or *q*) in order of frequency in English *writing*. ______
4. Using Appendix B in *AP* (p. 341), rank order, from most to least frequent, the alphabet letters for the stop consonants in order of frequency in English *speech*. ______
5. Using Appendix F in *AP* (p. 360), rank order the stop consonants from *least to most often misunderstood* in normal conversation. ______

6. Using the rankings that you obtained for questions 3, 4, and 5, compare the rankings for the *first three stops* in each answer.

   a. Do you think a general relation exists between writing, speaking, and intelligibility for the stops? (Circle) YES NO

   b. What do you think accounts for the closer relationship between speech and perception than writing? ____

B. Using Appendix B (p. 341) in *AP*, answer the following questions.

7. Rank the vowels /ɪ, ɛ, æ, ə, ɚ, o/ in terms of their frequency in *speech* by writing their phonetic symbols in the spaces provided. 1st ____ 2nd ____ 3rd ____ 4th ____ 5th ____ 6th ____. For all the vowel sounds, these six vowels account for what percent of use in *speech*? ________________

8. In order, what are the 10 most frequent sounds in American English *speech*? ________________

   ____

9. In order, what are the 10 least frequent sounds in American English *speech*? ________________

   ____

10. Now compare the rankings that you obtained for items 8 and 9 to answer these questions:

    a. Which set of rankings (8 or 9) is characterized by

       1. more alveolar sounds? ________________________________

       2. more +Distributed sounds? ________________________________

       3. more back sounds? ________________________________

       4. more front sounds? ________________________________

       5. more alveopalatal sounds? ________________________________

       6. more fricative sounds? ________________________________

    b. What conclusion can you reach about the phonetic features of those sounds that are most frequent in English speech?

       ____

       ____

C. Using Appendix F (p. 360) in *AP*, answer the following questions.

11. Refer to your answers for question 8 and rank order those sounds from *least to most frequently misunderstood* at normal conversational intensities in American English. Also include the percentage for each of the 10 sounds.

    ____

    ____

12. Do the same for the ranking that you obtained in question 9, again listing the sounds from *least to most frequently misunderstood* in American English at normal conversational intensities. Include the percentage for each of the 10 sounds.

    ____

    ____

13. What is the total percentage accounted for by each group?

    a. The most frequent sounds account for ________ percent of error.

    b. The least frequent sounds account for ________ percent of error.

c. The conclusion from this analysis is: ______________________________

____

14. What prediction would you make if you took only the consonants from the rankings in questions 8 and 9 and used Appendix C in *AP* to determine if more frequent sounds developed before the less frequent ones? ______________________________

Look to see if you are correct!

D. Using Appendix C (p. 344) in *AP*, answer the following questions.

15. At what age do 51% of children have mastery of /f/? ______ years
16. At what age do 51% of children have mastery of /v/? ______ years
17. At what age do 51% of children have mastery of /z/? ______ years
18. At what age do 51% of children have mastery of /ʒ/? ______ years

E. Using various appendixes in *AP*, what is the

19. strongest sound in American English? ______________________________
20. weakest sound in American English? ______________________________
21. most frequent sound in American English? ______________________________
22. most frequent grapheme in written English? ______________________________
23. least frequent phoneme in American English? ______________________________
24. least frequent grapheme in American English? ______________________________
25. most frequently misunderstood sound in American English? ______________________________
26. nasal phoneme that develops after the other nasals in child speech? ______________________________
27. most frequently used nasal phoneme in English speech? ______________________________

Review Exercise 14.7. Acoustic Descriptions of Sounds

Read Appendix D in *AP* (p. 350) and then answer these questions.

1. What is a wide-band spectrogram? ______________________________

____

2. What is a narrow-band spectrogram? ______________________________

____

3. Suppose that you are interested in studying intonation patterns in a language. What type of spectrogram would you use? ______________________________
4. Suppose you wanted to compare vowel resonances in speakers of German and Vietnamese. What type of spectrogram would serve this purpose? ______________________________
5. Compare the power spectra for the /s/ and the /ʃ/ (refer to pages 133 and 143 in *AP*) to answer the following true/false questions.

____ a. The concentration of energy in the frequency dimension for /s/ is higher than that for /ʃ/.

____ b. As a result, /s/ sounds lower in pitch than /ʃ/.

Review Exercise 14.8. Broad Transcription

Transcribe these proverbs using broad transcription.

1. The best way out is always through.

____

2. People who are late are often much jollier than the people who have to wait for them.

____

3. The only sure thing about luck is that it will change.

____

Review Exercise 4.9. Prosodic Transcription

Transcribe this limerick, paying special attention to stress-marker placement. Also show falling pitch.

A young phonetician named Rod. ____________________________

Transcribed in a way that was odd. ____________________________

One thing he would do ____________________________

That made teachers quite blue ____________________________

Was to substitute theta for yod. ____________________________

Review Exercise 14.10. Narrow Transcription

Transcribe these examples of daffy definitions using narrow transcription.

1. Sibilants: The phonemes produced by the children within the same family.

____

____

2. Distinctive Features: What phoneticians possess that make them different from other people.

____

____

____

3. Register: A place where students of phonetics keep their money.

____

____

References

Aesop's fables. (1947). New York: Grossett & Dunlap.

American heritage dictionary. (1985). Boston: Houghton Mifflin.

Chomsky, N., & Halle, M. (1968). *The sound pattern of English.* New York: Harper & Row.

Darley, F., Aronson, A., & Brown, J. (1975). *Motor speech disorders.* Philadelphia: W.B. Saunders.

Dewey, G. (1971). *English spelling: Roadblock to reading.* New York: Teachers College Press.

Duckworth, M., Allen, G., Hardcastle, W., & Ball, M. (1990). Extensions to the International Phonetic Alphabet for the transcription of atypical speech. *Clinical Linguistics & Phonetics, 4*(4), 273–280.

Jakobson, R., Fant, C. G. M., & Halle, M. (1952). *Preliminaries to speech analysis: The distinctive features and their correlates.* Cambridge, MA: The MIT Press.

Klatt, D. H. (1975). Voice onset time, friction, and aspiration in word-initial consonant clusters. *Journal of Speech and Hearing Research, 18*, 686–706.

Ladefoged, P. (1990). The revised International Phonetic Alphabet. *Language, 66*(3), 550–552.

Oxford American dictionary. (1980). New York: Avon.

Random House unabridged dictionary. (1987). (2nd ed.). New York: Random House.

Stern, D. A. (1987). *The sound & style of American English.* Los Angeles: Dialect Accent Specialists.

Webster's II, new Riverside dictionary. (1984). Boston: Houghton Mifflin.

Webster's new world dictionary. (1988). (3rd ed.). New York: World.

Webster's tenth new collegiate dictionary. (1993). Springfield, MA: Merriam-Webster.

Wise, C. M. (1957). *Applied phonetics.* Englewood Cliffs. NJ: Prentice-Hall.

APPENDIX A

Printed and Handwritten Symbols

Key Words: pet, bet, tab, dab, kale, gale, fan, van, thigh, thy, sip, zip, shop, measure, hiss, chop, job, moat, keep 'em, note, sudden, sing, baking, yes, we, road, load, people, heal, hill, way, bed, bad, bud, abode, herd, herder, Luke, look, boat, haul, lock, buy, how, boy, you

Printed Symbol	Key Word	Written Symbol	Key Word
/ p /	pɛt	p	pɛt
/ b /	bɛt	b	bɛt
/ t /	tæb	t	tæb
/ d /	dæb	d	dæb
/ k /	kel	k	kel
/ g /	gel	g	gel
/ f /	fæn	f	fæn
/ v /	væn	v	væn
/ θ /	θa͜ɪ	θ	θa͜ɪ
/ ð /	ða͜ɪ	ð	ða͜ɪ
/ s /	sɪp	s	sɪp
/ z /	zɪp	z	zɪp
/ ʃ /	ʃɑp	ʃ	ʃɑp
/ ʒ /	mɛʒɚ	ʒ	mɛʒɚ

Printed Symbol	Key Word	Written Symbol	Key Word
/ h /	hɪs	h	hɪs
/ tʃ /	tʃɑp	tʃ	tʃɑp
/ dʒ /	dʒɑb	dʒ	dʒɑb
/ m /	mot	m	mot
/ m̩ /	kipm̩	m̩	kipm̩
/ n /	not	n	not
/ n̩ /	sʌdn̩	n̩	sʌdn̩
/ ŋ /	sɪŋ	ŋ	sɪŋ
/ ŋ̩ /	bekŋ̩	ŋ̩	bekŋ̩
/ j /	jɛs	j	jɛs
/ w /	wi	w	wi
/ r /	rod	r	rod.
/ l /	lod	l	lod
/ l̩ /	pipl̩	l̩	pipl̩

Printed Symbol	Key Word	Written Symbol	Key Word	Printed Symbol	Key Word	Written Symbol	Key Word
/ i /	hil	i	hil	/ u /	luk	u	luk
/ ɪ /	hɪl	ɪ	hɪl	/ ʊ /	lʊk	ʊ	lʊk
/ e /	we	e	we	/ o /	bot	o	bot
/ ɛ /	bɛd	ɛ	bɛd	/ ɔ /	hɔl	ɔ	hɔl
/ æ /	bæd	æ	bæd	/ ɑ /	lɑk	a	lak
/ ʌ /	bʌd	ʌ	bʌd	/ a͜ɪ /	ba͜ɪ	a͜ɪ	ba͜ɪ
/ ə /	ə'bod	ə	ə'bod	/ a͜ʊ /	ha͜ʊ	a͜ʊ	ha͜ʊ
/ ɝ /	hɝd	ɝ	hɝd	/ ɔ͜ɪ /	bɔ͜ɪ	ɔ͜ɪ	bɔ͜ɪ
/ ɚ /	hɝdɚ	ɚ	hɝdɚ	/ j͜u /	j͜u	j͜u	j͜u

APPENDIX B

Selected Answers to Some Transcription Exercises

Part I

Transcription Exercise 2.5. Review

pit	pɪt	bad	bæd
cone	kon	mow	mo
gag	gæg	kin	kɪn
dough	do	dead	dɛd
dope	dop	act	ækt
cab	kæb	known	non
debt	dɛt	man	mæn
knack	næk	bid	bɪd
owe	o	net	nɛt
gap	gæp	lap	læp

Transcription Exercise 2.6. Introducing /ŋ/ as in ink

king	kɪŋ	gang	gæŋ
ink	ɪŋk	ping	pɪŋ
tank	tæŋk	bank	bæŋk
pink	pɪŋk	ding	dɪŋ
tang	tæŋ	bang	bæŋ

Transcription Exercise 2.7. Transcribing Words with /l/ and /r/

land	'lænd	plaque	'plæk
chrome	'krom	dread	'drɛd
rib	'rɪb	cling	'klɪŋ

roan	ˈron	rink	ˈrɪŋk
wreck	ˈrɛk	load	ˈlod
rill	ˈrɪl	pole	ˈpol
bring	ˈbrɪŋ	crib	ˈkrɪb
blown	ˈblon	drag	ˈdræg

Transcription Exercise 2.8. Practice With the Pitch Test, Marking Primary Stress, and Vowel Reduction With /ə/

Words Stressed on the First Syllable		Words Stressed on the Second Syllable	
Tampa	ˈtæmpə	abode	əˈbod
talcum	ˈtælkəm	amid	əˈmɪd
Alan	ˈælən	abet	əˈbɛt

Transcription Exercise 2.9. Reduced Vowels

cryptic	ˈkrɪptɪk	bandit	‘bændɪt
coma	ˈkomə	cabin	ˈkæbɪn
tannic	ˈtænɪk	boa	ˈboə
cobra	ˈkobrə	adept	ɑˈdɛpt
Mona	ˈmonə	delta	ˈdɛltə

Transcription Exercise 2.10. Practicing Transcribing / ɚ /

odor	ˈodɚ	glimmer	ˈglɪmɚ
erode	əˈrod ~ ɚˈod	broker	ˈbrokɚ
planner	ˈplænɚ	peppered	ˈpɛpɚd

Transcription Exercise 2.11d. Transcribing Words With Past Tense Endings

batted	ˈbætəd	knitted	ˈnɪtəd
bagged	ˈbægd	mapped	ˈmæpt
kidnaped	ˈkɪdnæpt	lagged	ˈlægd

Transcription Exercise 2.12. Review of Transcription Principles

editor	ˈɛd$\overset{ə}{ɪ}$tɚ	limited	ˈlɪm$\overset{ə\ ɪ}{ɪ}$təd
dragon	ˈdrægən	kidder	ˈkɪdɚ
moaned	ˈmond	owned	ˈond
trend	ˈtr$\overset{ɪ}{ɛ}$nd	pecked	ˈpɛkt
condone	kənˈdon	connected	kəˈnɛkt$\overset{ɪ}{ə}$d

Transcription Exercise 3.3. Transcribing the Syllabic Consonants

*tilt	tɪlt	redden	ˈrɛdn̩
middle	ˈmɪdl̩	wrinkle	ˈrɪŋkl̩

kettle	'kɛt̬ 'l̩	ogle	'ogl̩
mitten	'mɪtn̩	brittle	'brɪt̬l̩
*kelp	kɛlp	bitten	'bɪtn̩

Transcription Exercise 3.4. Using Syllabics in Informal Speech

	Formal Speech		Informal Speech
open	'opən		'opm̩
captain	'kæptən	"cap'n"	'kæpm̩
blacken	'blækən		'blækŋ̍
broken	'brokən		'brokŋ̍
napping	'næpɪŋ		'næpm̩

Transcription Exercise 3.7. The Loss of /t/ in Informal Speech

mental	ɪ 'mɛnl̩	planter	'plænɚ
memento	ɪ mə'mɛno	(to) contend	ɪ kən'tɛnd
planner	'plænɚ	pinto	'pɪno

Transcription Exercise 3.10. Transcribing /ŋ/

angle	'æŋgl̩	linking	'lɪŋkɪŋ
ringer	'rɪŋɚ	dangled	'dæŋgl̩d

Transcription Exercise 3.13. Review

canal	kə'næl	intellect	'ɪnəlɛkt
maddening	'mædn̩ɪŋ	Manila	mə'nɪlə
trampling	'træmplɪŋ~l̩	technical	'tɛknəkl̩
alpaca	æl'pækə	peppering	'pɛpɚɪŋ~ rɪŋ
Arabic	æ 'ɛrəbɪk	pimento	ɪ pə'mɛno

Transcription Exercise 4.4. Using /hw/

whelp	'hwɛlp	whim	'hwɪm
wet	'wɛt	where	'hwɛr

Transcription Exercise 4.9. R-dropping in Southern American Dialect

yearn	'jɜn	Merlin	'mɜlɪn ~ən
entered	'ɛnəd ~ 'ɪnəd	polar	'polə

Transcription Exercise 4.12. Words Containing /u/ and /j͜u/

tune	'tun	cartoon	kɑr'tun
cute	'kj͜ut	yew	'j͜u
nude	'nud	noodle	'nj͜u~ 'nudl̩

Transcription Exercise 4.13. Review Transcription

ha-ha	'hɑhɑ	herb	'ɝb
Curt	'kɝt	wad	'wɑd
young	'jʌŋ	pucker	'pʌkɚ
wand	'wɑnd	purr	'pɝ
her	'hɝ	a block	ə 'blɑk
her pen	hɚ'pɛᶦn	crumb	'krʌm

Transcription Exercise 5.1. Transcribing the Sibilants

zap	'zæp	garage	gə'rɑʒ ~ gɚ'ɑʒ
sipper	'sɪpɚ	treasure	'trɛʒɚ
whiz	'wiz~ 'hwɪz	ruts	'rʌts

Transcription Exercise 5.2. The Devoicing of / z̥ /

cones	'konz̥	cobwebs	'kɑbwɛbz̥
pose	'poz̥	runs	'rʌnz̥
buzz	'bʌz̥	snooze	'snuz̥

Transcription Exercise 5.3. Grammatical Markers

knocks	'nɑks	boxes	'bɑksəz̥ ~ ɪz̥
ceramics	sɚ'ræmɪks ~ sə	echoes	'ɛkoz̥
student's	'studn̩ts	bibs	'bɪbz̥
dishes	'dɪʃəz̥ ~ ɪz̥	mirages	mə'rɑʒəᶦz̥ ~ mɚ'ɑ
Tom's	'tɑmz̥	Alice's	'æləsəz̥ ~ sɪz̥

Transcription Exercise 5.4. Transcribing "ns" Combinations

sense	'sɛᶦnᵗs	scents	'sɛᶦnts
cents	'sɛᶦnts	insect	'ɪnsɛkt
mints	'mɪnts	mince	'mɪnᵗs

Transcription Exercise 5.5. Practice With /e/

aide	'ed	player	'pleɚ
eight	'et	nation	'neʃən ~ ɪn
paced	'pest	pest	'pɛst
attain	ə'ten	locate	'loket

Transcription Exercise 5.8. Practicing the /v/ to /b/ Shift

	Formal Speech	Informal (/'b, m̩/) Speech
driven	'drɪvən ~ ɪn	'drɪbm̩
eleven	ə'levən ~ ɪn	ə'lɛbm̩

Transcription Exercise 5.9. Transcribing /ʊ/

should	'ʃʊd	sugar	'ʃʊgɚ
booking	'bʊkɪŋ	shook	'ʃʊk
look	'lʊk	luck	'lʌk

Transcription Exercise 5.11. Transcribing /ɔ͜ɪ/

point	'pɔ͜ɪnt	boy	'bɔ͜ɪ
destroy	d$\overset{ə}{ɪ}$'strɔ͜ɪ	employ	$\overset{ɪ}{ɛ}$m'plɔ͜ɪ
alloy	'ælɔ͜ɪ	Roy	'rɔ͜ɪ

Transcription Exercise 5.12. Transcribing /a͜ɪ/

I	'a͜ɪ	sky	'ska͜ɪ
kind	'ka͜ɪnd	buy	'ba͜ɪ
mine	'ma͜ɪn	ride	'ra͜ɪd

Transcription Exercise 5.13. Practice Transcribing the Intrusive Schwa-Glide

wail	'we^{ə}l	pearl	'pɝ^{ə}l
mild	'ma͜ɪ^{ə}ld	pool	'pu^{ə}l
girl	'gɝ^{ə}l	coiled	'kɔ͜ɪ^{ə}ld
talc	'tælk	boiling	'bɔɪ^{ə}lɪŋ ~ ɔ͜ɪlɪŋ

Transcription Exercise 5.14. Dialect Variation and /a͜ɪ/

	General American	Southern American /a/
I	'a͜ɪ	'a
wise	'wa͜ɪz̥	'waz̥

Transcription Exercise 6.1. Transcribing /ɔ/

bought	'bɔt	brought	'brɔt
audible	'ɔdəbl̩	vaunt	'vɔnt
often	'ɔfən	sprawl	'sprɔl
fog	'fɔg	haul	'hɔl

Transcription Exercise 6.3. Contrasting /ɔ/ and /ɔ͜ɪ/

boil	'bɔɪl ~ ɔ͜ɪ^{ə}l	ball	'bɔl
loin	'lɔ͜ɪn	lawn	'lɔn

Transcription Exercise 6.4. Transcribing /ɔr/

score	'skɔr	born	'bɔrn
forward	'fɔrwɚd	organized	'ɔrgəna͜ɪzd

Transcription Exercise 6.6. Transcribing /i/

heat	ˈhit	heed	ˈhid
unbeatable	ənˈbit̬əbl̩	extreme	ɪkˈstrim
preschool	ˈpriskul ~ ᵊl	speed	ˈspid

Transcription Exercise 6.10. Transcribing /aʊ̯/

cloud	ˈklaʊ̯d	amounts	əˈmaʊ̯nts
town	ˈtaʊ̯n	cow	ˈkaʊ̯
flounder	ˈflaʊ̯ndɚ	sauerkrant	ˈsaʊ̯ɚˈkraʊ̯t

Transcription Exercise 6.11. Transcribing /θ/ and /ð/

there	ˈðɛr	thus	ˈðʌs
theft	ˈθɛft	thirst	ˈθɝst

Transcription Exercise 6.12. The Affricates

chime	ˈtʃaɪ̯m	church	ˈtʃɝtʃ
gent	ˈdʒɛ̃nt (ɪ above ɛ)	jinx	ˈdʒɪŋks
jammed	ˈdʒæmd	chamber	ˈtʃembɚ

Transcription Exercise 7.4. Deciding on Primary Stress in Words

Canadian	kəˈnediən (ɪ above ə)	introduction	ɪntrəˈdʌkʃən (ɪ above ə)
principle	ˈprɪn(t)səpl̩	optimistic	ɑptəˈmɪstɪk
embarrassment	ɛmˈbærəsmənt (ɪ above ɛ, ɛ above æ, ɪ above ə)	syllable	ˈsɪləbl̩

Transcription Exercise 7.5. Primary Stress in Short Phrases

the	ˈðʌ	the book	ðə ˈbʊk
a	ˈʌ ~ ˈe	a lot	ə ˈlɑt
in	ˈɪn	in the park	ɪn ðə ˈpɑrk

Transcription Exercise 7.9. Two Levels of Stress in Words

anthropology	ˈænθrəˈpɑlədʒi	exaggeration	ɪgˌzædʒɚˈeʃən (ɪ above ə)
apologetic	əˌpɑləˈdʒɛt̬ɪk	dilapidated	dəˈlæpəˌdet̬ɪd

Transcription Exercise 8.5. Devoicing of Liquids

grain	ˈgren	crane	ˈkr̥en
sprain	ˈspren	tractor	ˈtr̥æktɚ
placemat	ˈpl̥esmæt	bloodmobile	ˈblʌdmobiᵊl

Transcription Exercise 8.6d. Transcribing Various /l/ Allophones

linseed oil	ˈl̺ɪnsid ˈɔɪ̯ᵊɫ	calculator	ˈkæʟkjəl̺et̬ɚ
illegal	ɪˈl̺igʟ̩	linoleum	l̺ɪˈnol̺iəm

Part II

Transcription Exercise 9.3. Marking Short Phonological Phrases

To be or not to be, / that is the question. / Whether 'tis nobler in the mind / to suffer the slings and arrows / of outrageous fortune / or by opposing end them./

Transcription Exercise 11.1. Tensing of Lax Vowels

Mister Fox was just about famished and thirsty, too.

ˌmistɛr ˌfɑks wɑz ˈdʒust ebaʊ̯t ˌfemiʃt ænd ˈθɛrsti ˌtu

Transcription Exercise 11.2. Airflow on the Interdental Fricatives (Dentalization)

The thimbles that Thurman threw bothered father.

d̪ə ˈt̪ɪmbl̩z d̪æt̪ ‿t̪ mənˌt̪ru ˈbɑd̪ɚd ˌfɑd̪ɚ

Transcription Exercise 11.3. Wrong Placement of the Interdentals

The thimbles that Thurman threw bothered father.

zə ‘sɪmbl̩z‿z ætˌsɚmən ˌsru ˈbɑzɚd ˌfɑzɚ

Transcription Exercise 11.4a. Using /ɾ/ for /r/

The crimson roses grew over Farmer Ross's residence.

ðə ˈkɾɪmzən ˌɾozəz gɾu ovəɾ ˈfɑɾməɾ ˌɾ(ɾ)ɑsɪz ˌɾɛzədən^{t}s

Transcription Exercise 11.4b. Use of /l/ for /r/

The crimson roses grew over Farmer Ross's residence.

ðə ˈklɪmzən ˌlozəz ˌglu ovə ˈfɑmə ˌlɑs(ə)ɪz ˌlɛzəd(ɪ)ən^{t}s

Transcription Exercise 11.4c. Use of /v/ for /w/

We witnessed wigwams everywhere.

vi ˈvɪtnɪst ˌvɪgvɑmz ˈɛvrivɛr

Transcription Exercise 11.4d. Use of /s/ for /ʃ/

Shepherds should cautiously establish pawnshops.

‘sɛpɚdz̥ sʊd ˌkɒsəsli əˌstæblɪs ˌ pɒnsɑps

Transcription Exercise 11.4e. Use of /r/ for /ʒ/

Asia's unusual treasures gave visual pleasure.

ˌezəz ənˈjuzʊəl ˌtrɛzɚz ˌgev‿ˌvɪzʊəl ˌplɛzɚ

Transcription Exercise 12.1. Cluster Reduction

Please bring a clean spoon for the snack.

‘pɪz bɪŋ ə ˌkin ˌpun fɚ ðə ˈnæk

Transcription Exercise 12.2. Stopping

Susie and Van saw four sheep at the zoo.

ˈtudi ən ˌbæn ˌtɒ ˈpɔr ˌtip æt də ˌdu

Transcription Exercise 12.3. Prevocalic Voicing

Timmy took cookies to the party.

ˈt̬ɪmi ˌt̬ʊk ͜ ˌk̬ʊk̬iz t̬ə ðə ˈp̬ɑrt̬i

Transcription Exercise 12.4. Assimilation

Tommy smiled as he put the cup on the table.

ˈpɑmi ˌfma͜ɪld æz hi pʊp ðə pəp ɑn ðə ˌpebl̩

Transcription Exercise 12.5. Gliding

Larry ran around the long lake.

ˈwæwi ˌwæn əˌwa͜ʊnd͜ðə ˈwɑŋ ˌwek

Transcription Exercise 12.6. The Frontal Lisp

Sam's sister sells zinnias in summer.

ˈs̪əemz̪̥ s̪ɪs̪tɚ s̪ɛlz̪ ͜ ˌz̪ ɪniəz̪ ɪn s̪əmɚ

Transcription Exercise 12.7. The Lateral Lisp

Sam's sister sells zinnias in summer.

ˈl̥͜s əeml̥͜z l̥͜s ɪl̥͜s tɚ l̥͜s ɛl͜z l͜z ɪniəl͜z ɪn l̥͜s əmɚ

Transcription Exercise 12.8. Overuse of the Velar l

Floyd let Lyle list the syllables.

ˈfʟɔ͜ɪd ʟɛt ʟa͜ɪəʟ͜ʟɪst ðə ˈsɪʟəbəʟ̩z̥

APPENDIX C

Comparison of Commonly Used Phonetic Alphabets

Consonants

Sound Classes	IPA	AH	OA	RH	All Dictionaries	W2	WNW	W10C	Key Words
Voiceless stops	p				p				*p*a*p*er
	t				t				*t*icke*t*
	k				k				*k*ic*k*
Voiced stops	b				b				im*b*i*b*e
	d				d				*d*rea*d*
	g				g				*g*a*g*
Voiceless fricatives	f				f				*f*lu*ff*
	θ	th	th	t͜h		th	tħ	th	*th*in
	s				s				*s*au*c*e
	ʃ	sh	sh	s͜h		sh	sh	sh	fa*sh*ion
	h				h				*h*uff
Voiced fricatives	v				v				*v*al*v*e
	ð	*th*	*th*	*tħ*		*th*	th	t̲h̲	*th*en
	z				z				*z*oo*s*
	ʒ	zh	*zh*	z͜h		zh	zh	zh	lei*s*ure
Affricates	tʃ	ch	ch	c͜h		ch	ch	ch	*ch*ur*ch*
	dʒ				j				*j*u*dg*e
Nasals	m				m				*m*ada*m*
	m̩	—	—	—		—	—	ᵊm	"op*en*"
	n				n				*n*a*nn*y
	n̩	—	ăn, ĕn ĭn, ŏn, ŭn	ᵊn		n	'n	ᵊn	butt*on*
	ŋ	n	ng	n͡g		ng	ŋ	ŋ	*s*i*n*ki*ng*
	ŋ̩	ng	—	—		—	—	ᵊŋ	lock-*and*-key

(continued)

Consonants *(continued)*

Sound Classes	IPA	AH	OA	RH	All Dictionaries	W2	WNW	W10C	Key Words
Lateral	l				l				*l*u*ll*
	l̩	l	ă, ĕ, il ŏl, ŭl,	ᵊl		l	’l	ᵊl	batt*le*
Approximants	w				w				*w*itch
	j				y				*y*ellow
	r				r				*r*ea*r*

Vowels

Sound Classes	IPA	AH	OA	RH	All Dictionaries	W2	WNW	W10C	Key Words
Front vowels	i	ē	ee	ē		ē	ē	ē	fr*ee*ly
	ɪ	ĭ	i	i		ĭ	i	i	m*i*ss
	e	ā	ay	ā		ā	ā	ā	pl*ay*
	ɛ	ĕ	e	e		ĕ	e	e	t*e*st
	æ	a	a	a		ă	a	a	*a*pple
Central vowels	ʌ	ŭ	u	u		ŭ	u	ə	ab*o*ve
	ə	ə	ă, ĕ, ĭ ŏ, ŭ	ə		ə	ə	ə	*a*bove
	ɝ	ûr	ur	ûr		ûr	ʉr	ər	th*ir*st
	ɚ	ər	ăr, ĕr, ĭr ŏr, ŭr	ər		ər	ər	ər	moth*er*
Back vowels	u	o͞o	oo	o͞o		o͞o	o͞o	ü	bl*ue*
	ʊ	o͝o	uu	o͝o		oo	oo	ü	p*u*sh
	o	ō	oh	ō		ō	ō	ō	fl*oa*t
	ɔ	ô	ɑw	ô		ô	ô	ȯ	b*ou*ght
	ɑ	ɑ, ŏ	ah, o	ä, ŏ		ä, ŏ	ä	ä	f*a*ther, c*o*t
Diphthongs	a͜ɪ	ī	I	ī		ī	ī	ī	v*i*ce
	a͜ʊ	ou	ow	ou		ou	*ou*	au̇	d*ou*bt
	ɔ͜ɪ	oi	oi	oi		oi	*oi*	ȯi	j*oi*n
	j͜u	yo͞o	yoo	yo͞o		yo͞o	yo͞o	yü	f*u*se

KEY:

IPA	Alphabet of the International Phonetic Association as used in this workbook.
AH	*American Heritage Dictionary*, 1985.
OA	*Oxford American Dictionary*, 1980.
RH	*Random House Unabridged Dictionary* (2nd ed.), 1987.
W2	*Webster's II, New Riverside Dictionary*, 1984.
WNW	*Webster's New World Dictionary* (3rd ed.), 1988.
W10C	*Merriam-Webster's Collegiate Dictionary, Tenth Edition*, 1993.

Index

5

k

6

g

20

ŋ

7

f

8

v

9

θ

10

ð

13

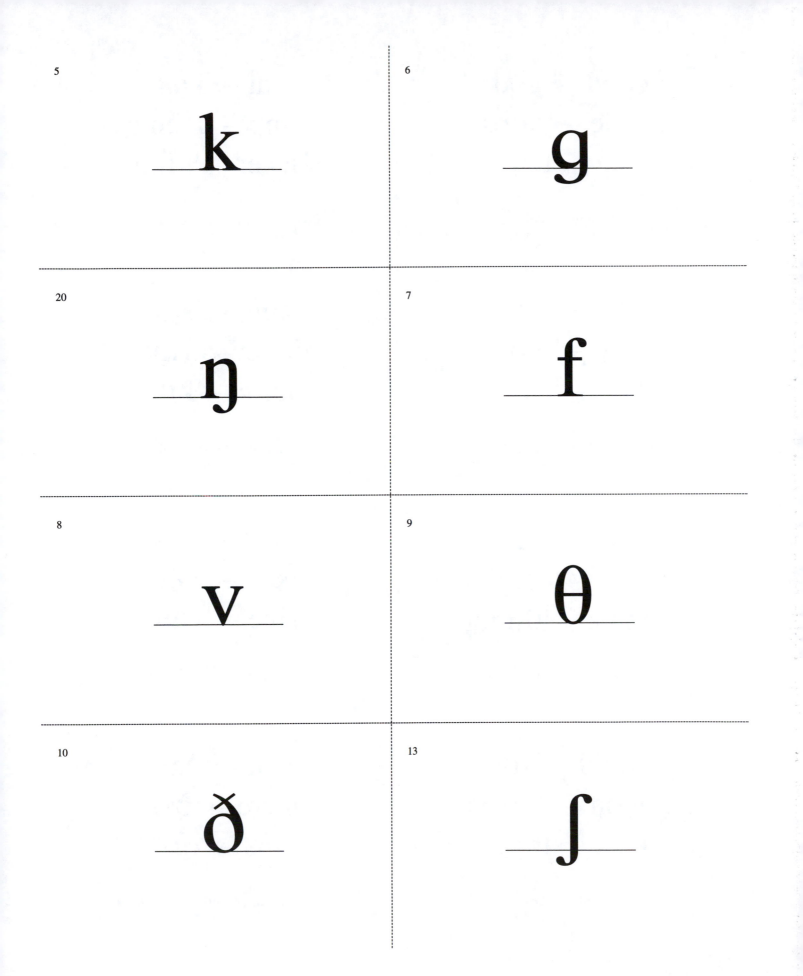

ʃ

6

*g*ood – ˈgʊd

*g*ar*g*le – ˈgɑrgl̩

be*g* – ˈbɛg

Voiced (Lingua-) Velar Stop

5

*c*at – ˈkæt

*c*amp – ˈkæmp

*k*ic*k*er – ˈkɪkɚ

Voiceless (Lingua-) Velar Stop

7

*f*our – ˈfɔr

*f*ly – ˈfla͜ɪ

hal*f* – ˈhæf

Voiceless Labiodental Fricative

20

si*ng* – ˈsɪŋ

ri*ng*er – ˈrɪŋɚ

ki*ng* – ˈkɪŋ

Voiced Velar Nasal
the "eng"

9

*th*irty – ˈθɝt̬i

*th*ank – ˈθæŋk

*th*imble – ˈθɪmbl̩

Voiced Interdental Fricative
the "theta"

8

*v*ase – ˈves

*v*ery – ˈvɛri

*v*ine – ˈva͜ɪn

Voiced Labiodental Fricative

13

*sh*ould – ˈʃʊd

fa*sh*ion – ˈfæʃən

tra*sh* – ˈtræʃ

Voiceless (Lingua-) Palatal (Grooved) Fricative
the "esh"

10

*th*at – ˈðæt

*th*ere – ˈðɛr

*th*is – ˈðɪs

Voiced Interdental Fricative
the "eth"

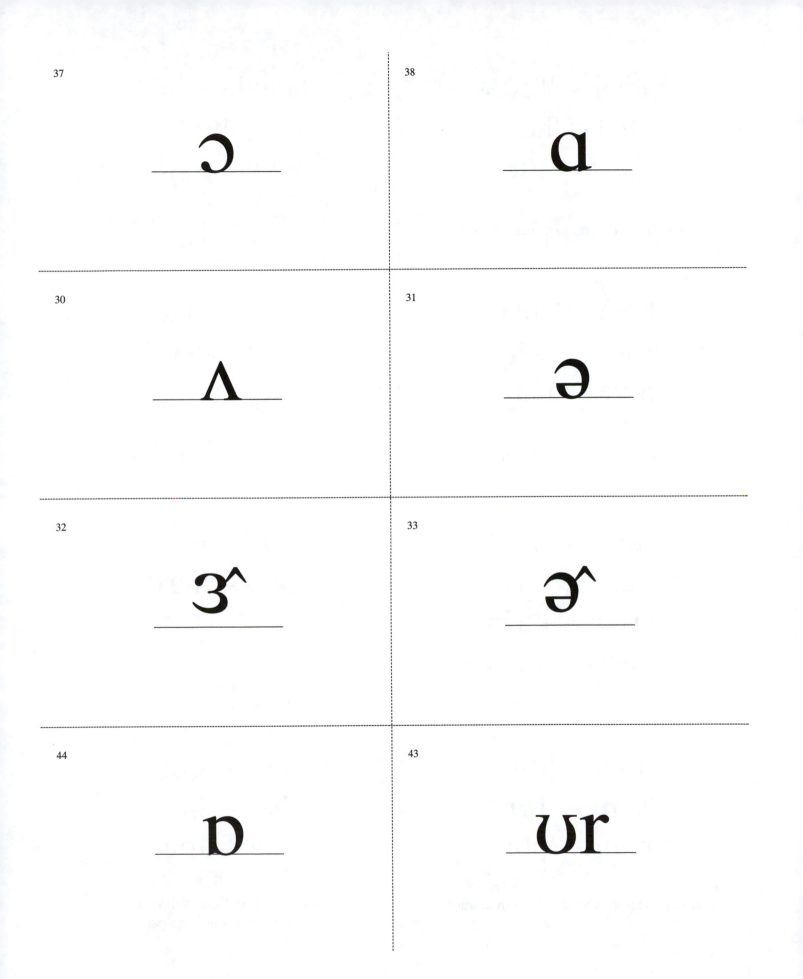

37 ɔ	38 ɑ
30 ʌ	31 ə
32 ɝ	33 ɚ
44 ɒ	43 ʊr

38

*fa*ther – ˈfɑðɚ

h*o*t – ˈhɑt

l*o*ck – ˈlɑk

Low Back Lax (Unrounded) Vowel

37

b*ou*ght – ˈbɔt

c*au*ght – ˈkɔt

t*au*ght – ˈtɔt

Low Mid Back Lax Rounded Vowel
the "open-o"

31

*a*bout – əˈba͡ʊt

All*e*n – ˈælən

*a*live – əˈla͡ɪv

Mid-Central Lax
(Unstressed) (Unrounded) Neutral Vowel
the "schwa"

30

b*u*d – ˈbʌd

h*u*t – ˈhʌt

*u*p – ˈʌp

Lower Mid-Central-to-Back Lax
(Unrounded) Neutral Vowel
the "caret"

33

moth*er* – ˈmʌðɚ

herd*er* – ˈhɝdɚ

curl*er* – ˈkɝlɚ

Mid-Central /r/-colored Lax Vowel
(Unstressed)
the "unstressed schwar"

32

b*ir*d – bɝd

h*er*d – ˈhɝd

c*ur*d – ˈkɝd

Mid-central /r/-colored Tense
Vowel (Stressed)
the "stressed schwar"

43

to*ur* – ˈtʊr

s*ure* – ˈʃʊr

po*or* – ˈpʊr

A non-phonemic vowel + /r/ combination

44

g*o*t – ˈgɒt

h*o*t – ˈhɒt

l*o*g – ˈlɒg

Low Back Lax Rounded Vowel
(phonemic in some dialects)

14 ʒ	16 tʃ
17 dʒ	11 s
12 z	24 l
23 r	21 j

16

*ch*air – ˈtʃɛr
*ch*ur*ch* – ˈtʃɝtʃ
hi*tch* – ˈhɪtʃ

Voiceless Alveopalatal Affricate

14

trea*s*ure – ˈtrɛʒɚ
mea*s*ure – ˈmɛʒɚ
plea*s*ure – ˈplɛʒɚ

Voiced (Lingua-) Palatal (Grooved) Fricative
the "ezh"

11

*s*top – ˈstɑp
*s*issy – ˈsɪsi
ant*s* – ˈænts

Voiceless (Lingua-) Alveolar (Grooved) Fricative

17

bri*dg*e – ˈbrɪdʒ
*j*am – ˈdʒæm
*g*em – ˈdʒɛm

Voiced Alveopalatal Affricate

24

*l*ate – ˈlet
ye*ll*ow – ˈjɛlo
*s*amp*l*e – ˈsæmpl̩

Voiced (Alveolar) Lateral (Liquid)

12

*z*ebra – ˈzibrə
bu*zz*er – ˈbʌzɚ
*z*oo – ˈzu

Voiced (Lingua-) Alveolar (Grooved) Fricative

21

*y*ellow – ˈjɛlo
*y*am – ˈjæm
back*y*ard – bækˈjɑrd

Voiced (Lingua-) Palatal (On-) Glide
(Semivowel)
the "yod"

23

*r*ide – ˈraɪ̯d
a*r*ose – əˈroz
ca*r* – ˈkɑr

Voiced Alveo-Palatal Liquid (Glide)
(Semivowel)

15

h

22

w

18

m

1

p

2

b

3

t

4

d

19

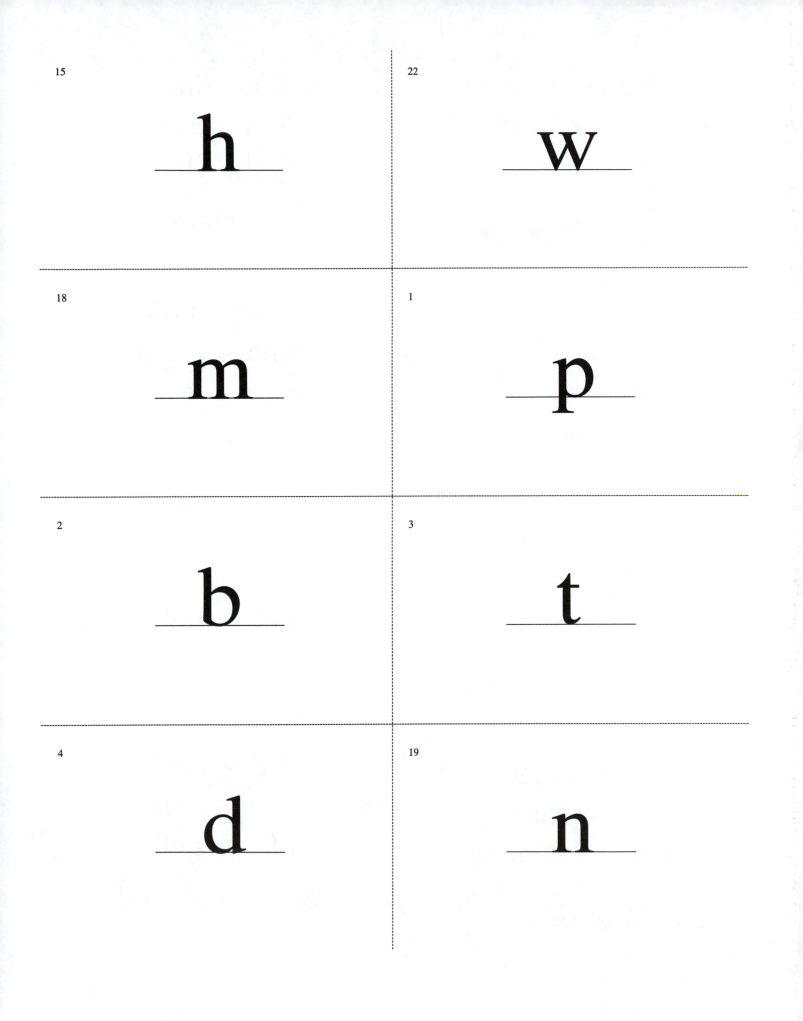

n

22

*w*agon – ˈwæɡən

t*w*in – ˈtwɪn

*w*ine – ˈwa͜ɪn

Voiced Bilabial (Lingua-Velar)
(On-) Glide (Semivowel)

15

*h*ot – ˈhɑt

*h*ow – ˈha͜ʊ

*h*igh – ˈha͜ɪ

Voiceless Glottal Fricative

1

*p*op – ˈpɑp

*p*lant – ˈplænt

a*pp*le – ˈæpl̩

Voiceless Bilabial Stop

18

*m*o*m* – ˈmɑm

*m*ine – ˈma͜ɪn

A*m*y – ˈemi

Voiced Bilabial Nasal

3

*t*o*t*e – ˈtot

*t*ime – ˈta͜ɪm

*t*ell – ˈtɛl

Voiceless (Lingua-) Alveolar Stop

2

*b*oy – ˈbɔ͜ɪ

*b*at – ˈbæt

*b*o*b* – ˈbɑb

Voiced Bilabial Stop

19

*n*ow – ˈna͜ʊ

*n*oo*n* – ˈnun

a*n*imal – ˈænəml̩

Voiced (Lingua-) Alveolar Nasal

4

*d*a*d* – ˈdæd

*d*ime – ˈda͜ɪm

i*d*le – ˈa͜ɪdl̩

Voiced (Lingua-) Alveolar Stop

39

aɪ͜

40

aʊ͜

41

ɔɪ͜

42

ju͜

45

ɔr

46

ɑr

48

ɛr

47

ir

40

how – ˈha͜ʊ

cow – ˈka͜ʊ

now – ˈna͜ʊ

Rising Low Front to High Back
(Offglide) Diphthong

39

I – ˈa͜ɪ

sky – ˈska͜ɪ

try – ˈtra͜ɪ

Rising Low Front to High Front
(Offglide) Diphthong

42

you – ˈj͜u

cue – ˈkj͜u

few – ˈfj͜u

High Front to High Back
(Onglide) Diphthong

41

boy – ˈbɔ͜ɪ

toy – ˈtɔ͜ɪ

Roy – ˈrɔ͜ɪ

Rising Mid Back to High Front
(Offglide) Diphthong

46

are – ˈɑr

car – ˈkɑr

bar – ˈbɑr

A non-phonemic vowel + /r/ combination

45

door – ˈdɔr

bore – ˈbɔr

score – ˈskɔr

A non-phonemic vowel + /r/ combination

47

ear – ˈir

fear – ˈfir

near – ˈnir

A non-phonemic vowel + /r/ combination

48

hair – ˈhɛr

bare – ˈbɛr

fair – ˈfɛr

A non-phonemic vowel + /r/ combination

25

i

26

ɪ

27

e

28

ɛ

29

æ

34

u

35

ʊ

36

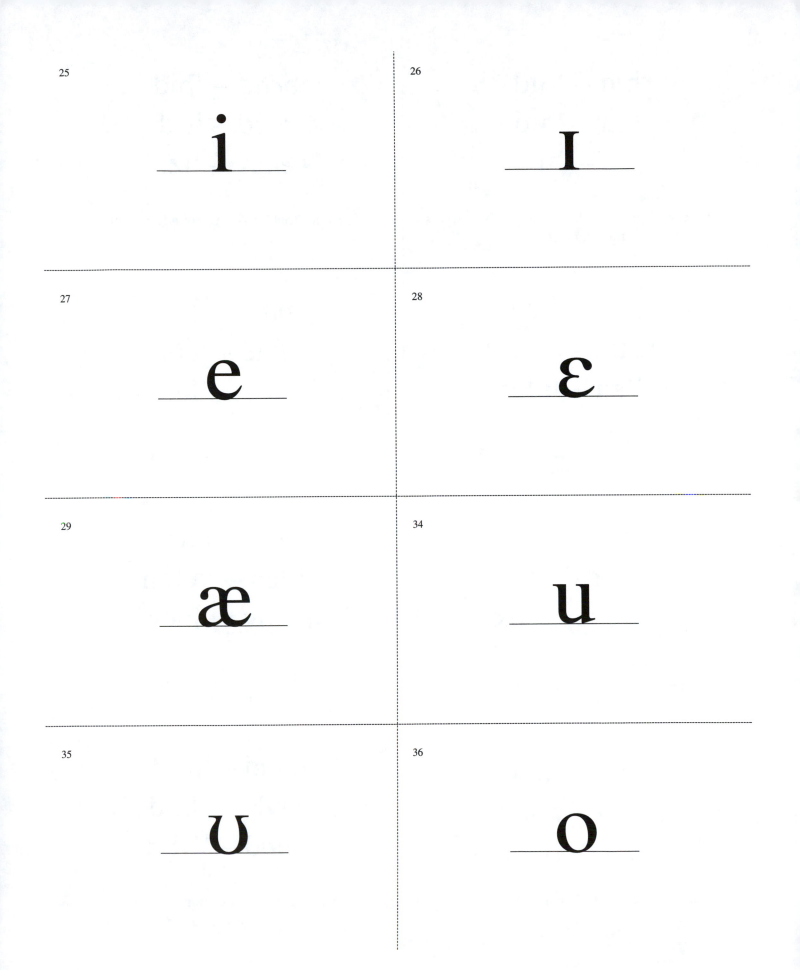

o

26

b*i*d – ˈbɪd

h*i*d – ˈhɪd

*i*f – ˈɪf

(Lower) High Front Lax (Unround) Vowel
the “capped-*i*”

25

b*ea*d – ˈbid

r*ea*d – ˈrid

*ea*sy – ˈizi

High Front Tense (Unround) Vowel

28

b*e*d – ˈbɛd

h*ea*d – ˈhɛd

*E*llen – ˈɛlən

(Lower) Mid Front Lax (Unround) Vowel
the “epsilon”

27

b*ai*t – ˈbet

*a*ble – ˈebl̩

l*a*te – ˈlet

Mid Front Tense (Unround) Vowel

34

b*oo*t – ˈbut

r*oo*ster – ˈrustɚ

l*oo*ps – ˈlups

High Back Tense (Rounded) Vowel

29

h*a*t – ˈhæt

*A*llen – ˈælən

h*a*ppy – ˈhæpi

Low Front Lax (Unround) Vowel
the “ash”

36

b*oa*t – ˈbot

al*o*ne – əˈlon

*o*pen – ˈopən

Mid Back Tense (Rounded) Vowel

35

h*oo*d – ˈhʊd

c*ou*ld – ˈkʊd

w*oo*d – ˈwʊd

High Back Lax (Rounded) Vowel
the “flying-*u*”

Audio CDs to Accompany *Applied Phonetics Workbook,* Third Edition

ISBN 0-7693-0261-0

Computer CD Player Instructions

1. Insert the disk into the CD-ROM player of your computer.
2. The media player should automatically start and bring up track 1.
3. Use the media player as directed by the manufacturer.

For Windows: If the media player does not start automatically:

1. From the Start Menu, choose Programs, then Accessories.
2. Choose Entertainment or Multimedia, then a media player such as Windows® Media Player.
3. Browse to your CD-ROM drive and open the audio file you wish to play.

For Macintosh: If the media player does not start automatically:

1. Start the Apple CD Player.
2. Browse to your CD-ROM drive and open the audio file you wish to play.

System Requirements

- Audio CD player **or**
- Computer with double-spin CD-ROM drive, sound card, speakers or headphones, and media player software.